Lecture Notes in Medical Informatics

Vol. 1: Medical Informatics Europe 78. Proceedings 1978. Edited by J. Anderson. XI, 822 pages. 1978.

Vol. 2: D. Fenna, S. Abrahamsson, S. O. Lööw and H. Peterson, The Stockholm County Medical Information System. VI, 163 pages. 1978.

Vol. 3: Long-Term Studies on Side-Effects of Contraception – State and Planning. Symposium 1977. Edited by U. Kellhammer and K. Überla. VI, 240 pages. 1978.

Vol. 4: Clinical Trials in 'Early' Breast Cancer. Proceedings 1978. Edited by H. R. Scheurlen, G. Weckesser and I. Armbruster. VI, 283 pages. 1979.

Vol. 5: Medical Informatics Berlin 1979. Proceedings 1979. Edited by B. Barber, F. Grémy, K. Überla and G. Wagner. XXIII, 970 pages. 1979.

Vol. 6: Health Care Technology Evaluation. Proceedings, 1978. Edited by J. Goldman. VII, 118 pages. 1979.

Vol. 7: Technology and Health: Man and his World. Proceedings, 1978. Edited by G. Wagner, P. L. Reichertz and E. Masè. VI, 243 pages. 1980.

Vol. 8: Mathematical Aspects of Computerized Tomography. Proceedings 1980. Edited by F. Natterer. VIII, 309 pages. 1981.

Vol. 9: Computers and Mathematical Models in Medicine. Proceedings, 1977. Edited by D. Cardús and C. Vallbona. VIII, 315 pages. 1981.

Vol. 10: B. Fries, Applications of Operations Research to Health Care Delivery Systems. V, 107 pages. 1981.

Vol. 11: Medical Informatics Europe 81. Proceedings 1981. Edited by F. Grémy, P. Degoulet, B. Barber, and R. Salamon. XXIII, 975 pages. 1981.

Vol. 12: G. Wiederhold, Databases for Health Care. VI, 75 pages. 1981.

Vol. 13: The Computer and Blood Banking. Proceedings, 1981. Edited by J. R. Möhr and A. Kluge. X, 275 pages. 1981.

Vol. 14.: F. Wingert, Medical Informatics. X, 247 pages. 1981.

Vol. 15: Digital Image Processing in Medicine. Proceedings 1981. Edited by K. H. Höhne. VIII, 197 pages. 1981.

Vol. 16: Medical Informatics Europe 82. Proceedings, 1982. Edited by R.R. O'Moore, B. Barber, P.L. Reichertz, and F. Roger. XX, 938 pages. 1982.

Vol. 17: Biomedical Images and Computers. Proceedings, 1980. Edited by J. Sklansky and J.-C. Bisconte. VII, 332 pages. 1982.

Vol. 18: D.P. Pretschner, Engymetry and Personal Computing in Nuclear Medicine. V, 129 pages. 1982.

Vol. 19: R.L. Blum, Discovery and Representation of Causal Relationships from a Large Time-Oriented Clinical Database: The RX Project. XIX, 242 pages. 1982.

Vol. 20: S. Biefang, W. Köpcke, M.A. Schreiber, Manual for the Planning and Implementation of Therapeutic Studies. V, 100 pages. 1983.

Vol. 21: Influence of Economic Instability on Health. Proceedings, 1981. Edited by J. John, D. Schwefel, and H. Zöllner. VIII, 528 pages. 1983.

Vol. 22: Objective Medical Decision-making; Systems Approach in Acute Disease. Proceedings, 1983. Edited by J. E. W. Beneken and S. M. Lavelle. VIII, 243 pages. 1983.

Lecture Notes in Medical Informatics

Edited by P. L. Reichertz and D. A. B. Lindberg

32

Glenn D. Rennels

A Computational Model of Reasoning from the Clinical Literature

Springer-Verlag
Berlin Heidelberg New York London Paris Tokyo

Author

Glenn D. Rennels, M. D., Ph. D.
Medical Information Sciences Program
Stanford University, Medical School Office Building
Stanford, CA 94305 – 5479, USA

ISBN-13: 978-3-540-17949-8 e-ISBN-13: 978-3-642-93363-9
DOI: 10.1007/978-3-642-93363-9

2127/3140-543210

Foreword

As research on expert systems has moved well into its second decade, it has become popular to cite the limitations of the phenomenologic or associational approach to knowledge representation that was typical of first generation systems. For example, the Internist-1 knowledge base represents explicitly over 600 diseases, encoding associated disease manifestations (signs, symptoms, physical findings, and lab abnormalities) but failing to deal with the *reasons* that those findings may be present in the disease [Miller, R. A. 82]. In recent years Pople has sought to add detailed causal models to the knowledge base in a revised version of the program known as CADUCEUS [Pople 82]. Similarly, a typical production rule in the MYCIN system states inferences that may be drawn when specific conditions are found to be true [Buchanan 84], but the underlying explanations for such relationships are not encoded. Clancey has argued that MYCIN needs such "supporting knowledge" represented, especially if its knowledge base is to be used for teaching purposes [Clancey 83].

By the late 1970s, artificial intelligence researchers were beginning to experiment with reasoning systems that used detailed mechanistic or causal models of the object being analyzed. Among the best early examples were a program to teach students how to analyze electronic circuits [Brown 82] and a system for diagnosing problems with mechanical devices [Rieger 76]. Such developments were not lost on the medical expert system community, and by the early 1980s we were beginning to see systems that analyzed medical problems based on detailed symbolic models of pathophysiology [Patil 81].

At about this time Glenn Rennels, a physician who had interrupted post-graduate medical training to obtain a degree in Medical Information Sciences at Stanford, was beginning to search for a Ph.D. dissertation topic. Impressed though he was in the exploratory work using medical causal models of pathophysiology, his medical training and experience persuaded him that the approach would be applicable to only a small percentage of the clinical problems that beset physicians in practice. When he observed consultants giving advice in clinics or on the wards, only occasionally did he notice that mechanistic explanations were a key element of the analysis. More typically the experts would cite the literature, mentioning data from clinical trials that were judged pertinent to the question at hand. Even more importantly, it was clear that for many areas of medicine our understanding of pathophysiologic details is so limited that it would be *misleading* to use a mechanistic model, rather than empiric data from well-controlled studies, to guide decision making.

The management of primary breast cancer is a particularly good example of this latter point. Although physicians have a superficial model of disease progression and spread via the blood or lymphatics, those models have proved inappropriate and hence useless for therapeutic decision making. Instead it is a careful analysis of studies reported in the literature, with expertise in statistical interpretation and matching of patient populations, which is the basis for selecting therapy for breast cancer. Even so, there is ample opportunity for disagreement, as the ongoing controversy regarding alternative surgical approaches and the role of adjuvant radiotherapy reveals.

The Roundsman system subsequently developed by Rennels is a novel and clever effort to develop a consultant program that gives advice based on an explicit representation of the content of articles from the clinical literature. Rather than seeking a mechanistic explanation of observed phenomena, Roundsman must select the studies that are relevant to a specific question, isolate the pertinent data for the population of patients best matched to the current case, and then generate advice in the form of free text that is understandable, tactful, and persuasive. Rennels' success in this effort is the subject of the current volume. Although the system is specific to breast cancer management at present (due to the generous collaboration of an eminent oncologist, Dr. Frank Stockdale), the approach is general and should be broadly applicable in other medical domains where empirical data are the cornerstone of expert decision making (for example, the management of hyperlipoproteinemia).

Rennels' work on this project has been a source of considerable excitement for me. Glenn is the first doctoral graduate from a novel interdisciplinary degree program in Medical Information Sciences that we began in 1982. Sitting as it does at the interface between computer science, clinical medicine, biostatistics, and artificial intelligence, Roundsman is in the best tradition of high quality interdisciplinary research. It helps show, by example, the unique confluence of scholarly activities that help define medical informatics as a distinct emerging academic discipline. I will not soon forget the gratifying discussion after Glenn's Ph.D. oral examination when the other members of his examination committee (a computer scientist, biostatistician, and internist) each acknowledged that the work was original and fully worthy of the doctorate although none felt the scope, content, and emphasis would have matched precisely with the advanced degree requirements of their own department.

I accordingly commend to you this excellent book. Roundsman is good computer science, offering an impressive synthesis of recent ideas regarding object centered programming, statistical reasoning, heuristic problem solving, and text generation. It is also good medicine, showing how domain knowledge evolves over time and addressing important issues of how medical experts must integrate new knowledge and data with what they already know. But, perhaps most importantly, it is superb medical informatics and is accordingly a worthy addition to this influential series of research notes.

Edward H. Shortliffe

Palo Alto

March 1987

Acknowledgments

This work was supported in part by training grant LM-07033 from the National Library of Medicine and ONR contract N00014-81-K-0004. Computing resources have been provided by the Biomedical Research Technology Program under grant RR-00785 and by the Hewlett-Packard Company.

The research described in this book was possible only with the help of many colleagues and friends. I am especially grateful to Ted Shortliffe, Frank Stockdale, Perry Miller, and Brad Efron.

Portions of this work have been published or are in press in the *Encyclopedia of Artificial Intelligence* [Rennels 87a], *Medical Decision Making* [Rennels 87b], *Computer Methods and Programs in Biomedicine* [Rennels 87c], *Proceedings of the Fifth World Congress on Medical Informatics* [Rennels 86a], *Proceedings of the AAMSI Congress 86* [Rennels 86b], *Proceedings of the Tenth Annual Symposium on Computer Applications in Medical Care* [Rennels 86c], and the *Proceedings of the AAMSI Congress 87* [Rennels 86d].

Table of Contents

Table of Contents

Table of Contents

List of Figures

List of Tables

Chapter 1
Introduction

This book explores the premise that the clinical literature can, and should, play a central role in computer-based decision support. Specifically, the motivation underlying this research includes the following propositions:

- Reasoning from experimental evidence contained in the clinical literature is central to the decisions a physician makes in patient care.

- A computational model of that reasoning process, based upon a declarative representation for published reports of clinical studies, can drive a computer program that selectively tailors knowledge of the clinical literature as it applies to a particular case.

- The development of such a computational model may help us better understand the general principles of reasoning from experimental evidence both in medicine and in other appropriate domains.

The computer program described in this book is a novel type of medical advice system: its advice is based on the experimental evidence of published biostatistical reports rather than causal models. Biomedicine and the social sciences will repeatedly present problem domains for which reliable causal models do not yet exist, and in which reasoning from experimental evidence is central to optimal problem-solving.

1.1. Introduction to the Problem

Artificial intelligence research has increasingly emphasized the advantages of representing more fundamental knowledge about the problem domain than, for instance, a set of weighted links between observable findings and diagnostic hypotheses. Much of this work seeks to flesh out the *causal models* underlying *diagnostic* reasoning, and to represent those models ("deep models") in an expert system to help drive its reasoning process. For example, an electronic circuit or the human body is modelled, and computer programs are designed to search for causal explanations of malfunction [Patil 81, Davis 84, Genesereth 84]. Planning medical *management* has not been as fully investigated, but several projects are currently exploring the notion that causal models of human pathophysiology can drive the analysis of medical management, for instance by simulating the effects of perturbing homeostasis in different ways [Long 84].

When these models mirror a manufactured device (e.g., an electronic circuit) causal models may indeed provide a sound basis for advice systems. In empirical sciences such as biomedicine however, these models are secondary constructions, derived from experimental evidence. A medical example is breast cancer. Biological models of breast cancer are an unreliable basis for therapy planning and the physician's reasoning must be directly grounded in the primary sources of experimental evidence (clinical trial publications). The causal models are too simplistic for decisions about individual patients, so physicians use the empiric evidence from clinical studies.

This crucial partnership between medical practice and the published reports of clinical studies exists not just in oncology (e.g., breast cancer) but throughout a wide variety of medical specialties:

- A publication by McCarron challenges the theoretical basis of current hypertension treatment [McCarron 84]. The results of this study indict calcium deficiency, rather than sodium excess (the traditional putative cause) as being responsible for hypertension. The medical profession awaits more definitive clinical studies [Kolata 84].

- Clofibrate, a drug which lowers serum cholesterol levels, was a widely-used agent for prevention of ischemic heart disease until a randomized clinical trial [Oliver 78] showed that, although it appeared to prevent ischemic heart disease, it *increased* overall mortality by 25 percent. The mechanism of the apparently harmful effect of the drug is unknown [Oliver 84].

- Although physicians have for decades treated diabetic patients according to a goal of normalizing their blood glucose level, there is meager evidence that this therapy prevents the eye, kidney or heart damage associated with diabetes. In fact, the largest clinical trial on this subject [KROC 84] suggested that normalizing blood glucose does more harm than good.

- The treatment of choice for shock has for some time included high doses of corticosteroids, given early in the course of illness. Their beneficial effect was thought to be related primarily to their stabilizing action on cellular membranes, which had been demonstrated in vitro. Recently published reports of clinical research performed in Miami [Sprung 84] and in Dallas [Weigelt 85] offer firm evidence that corticosteroids have no effect on the survival of patients with shock, and have the negative effect of predisposing to infections.

Clinical trials might therefore be seen to represent the basic science of medical management. Seen in this light, it is not suprising that statistical techniques assume a central role in medical journals. For example, "Statistics in Practice" has been a featured section of the *New England Journal of Medicine* [Lavori 83, Bailar 84a], the *Mayo Clinic Proceedings* carried a twelve-part series on "Statistics for Clinicians" [O'Brien 81] and the *Annals of Internal Medicine* published a four-part series acknowledging the explosive increase in attention given to clinical trials [Feinstein 83].

Clinicians are well aware that good medical practice depends on keeping up-to-date with the clinical literature. A useful assessment of these publications goes far beyond mere reporting of statistical results. To use this literature most effectively, a physician must critically assess these studies in the context of a *particular patient*, and decide in what ways the experimental trial is relevant to the case at hand. Indeed, this very skill of recalling the key studies and evaluating how well those results apply to the patient is a process learned and practiced every day by teams of medical students and residents on "rounds". A computer system which fails to use this fundamental knowledge may therefore not fully capture the decision making process central to many medical domains. Nevertheless, there has been little or no research into the design of computer systems which reason explicitly from representations of clinical studies to provide decision support for physicians.

A goal of this research is to model the process of reasoning from the clinical trials literature. There are many medical domains in which such reasoning dominates. It is therefore important to explore how a machine might assist a clinician in this literature-based reasoning process. This book describes a computer program, named Roundsman, which draws upon structured representations of the clinical literature to critique plans for medical management.

The Roundsman project therefore contributes a model of medical decision making, but it differs substantially from causal modeling in that there is no desire to model a "device" and its function, but rather to model the structure of experimental evidence and its interpretation for decision-making. In medical terms, it is not pathophysiological knowledge which is represented, but knowledge about experimental trials and their relevance to a particular patient's management.

1.2. Research Themes

In Roundsman, a number of research themes were addressed. These are summarized here and discussed in more detail in the remainder of the book.

Modeling Distance From Study to Clinical Decision

In order to be useful clinically, a medical advice system that draws on biostatistical literature must have a mechanism for interpreting the applicability of the study to a specific clinical decision. For example, methodological flaws may weaken the strength of the conclusions, making the study less useful to the physician. Also, there is seldom a perfect match between the study population and the patient, or between the study's treatment protocol and the decision options that the clinician faces. It is unrealistic to disregard studies which are methodologically flawed or do not precisely fit the clinical question. Virtually all clinical studies have some methodological weakness, and if clinicians used only studies that perfectly matched their clinical questions they would rarely find even one such study. So the question becomes: to what degree and *for what reasons* are the conclusions weakened by these mismatches, and how do these mismatches affect the applicability of the study to a particular clinical decision? In summary, a representation for the study must be structured so that the computer can dynamically assess the relationship between the context of the study and the context of the particular decision which a physician faces.

It is one thing to develop numerical approximations for the "distance" from a study to the specific management decision facing a clinician. It is another to develop a medical advice system that can articulate the details of the distance assessment. It is unlikely that the results of the algorithm will serve as more than a source of insight to the user. Conveying the semantics of both the *clinical* and *biostatistical* considerations involved is the central goal of Roundsman's design. This goal requires that the representation be rich enough to classify important types of 1) methodological weaknesses, 2) mismatches between populations and patients, and 3) mismatches between study protocols and treatments. The semantics of these details must be captured in order to offer an insightful critique to the physicians who are users of the program.

Choosing Treatment and Explaining the Choice

Users of advice systems for medical management can be expected to demand a reasoned argument for the system's choice. A model of medical management should therefore be able to deal with both choice *and* explanation. Because of this need to model explanation as well as choice, a system builder may find that a *general theory* for selecting optimal treatment (e.g., the axioms of utility theory) may not be the best solution to use for a specific domain. Modeling a particular treatment decision frequently does not need the full power of a general approach. Furthermore, by tailoring a general technique to a particular domain in a restricted form it may be possible to better capture the character of the domain and allow choice and explanation to be more naturally modeled. On the other hand, a domain must be studied carefully to determine which restricted form(s) might be appropriate, and it is the power of the general theory that provides the means to express assumptions being made when employing a restricted form.

Interactions Between Studies

Even if applicability of single studies to a patient can be assessed, there remains a problem of representing and using a substantial body of *inter-study* relationships. For example, new research reports often cast previous reports in a new light, altering their interpretation. Consequently, when new studies are added to a system such as Roundsman there are new issues of interpretation which derive from the interactions between studies.

Inter-study relationships are important also when research results are in conflict. That is, there may be situations in which the results of different studies seem to imply different conclusions. The problem of resolving conflicts between studies is sometimes called "meta-analysis", and is currently an extremely active area of research in biostatistics.

1.3. The Roundsman System: Examples

The Roundsman system is a computer program based upon an abstract computational model of how a physician reasons from experimental evidence in the clinical literature. The computer program provides a useful artifact: the model's performance can be examined dynamically. Furthermore, by applying the system design to actual publications from medical journals, the adequacy of the model's ability to handle the demands of real-world literature can be better assessed.

Among the design goals established for the Roundsman computer program are the following:

1. Given a patient and a treatment proposal, the program must critique that decision by giving a reasoned analysis based on its knowledge of the literature.

2. The computer system's data structures must reflect a "publication-

centered" view as discussed in Chapter 3. In particular, the system's critique of a treatment proposal for a particular patient must spring from declarative representations of one or more studies' experimental design and observed outcomes.

3. There must be convenient ways to represent knowledge about the mismatches mentioned earlier (e.g., mismatches between the patient and the study population), many of which represent the subjective clinical judgments of our domain expert.

4. The details of these mismatches must influence system performance in a substantive and appropriate way.

5. The system must address clinical concerns in a realistic way, and produce an English prose analysis which is lucid enough that clinical practitioners and biostatisticians can evaluate the potential of this approach to decision support.

In most respects the Roundsman system meets these goals. To use Roundsman, the physician first describes his patient and proposes a therapy choice (see Fig. 1-1). Roundsman produces a prose critique of the plan in light of the relevant clinical studies. This critique is assembled dynamically, tailored to the particular patient, treatment decision and clinical study(ies).

Roundsman draws upon a "library" of clinical studies in order to gather information on the alternative treatment plans. The studies in Roundsman's library are not full-text copies of articles, but instead are high-level representations of the study's features. The system makes conclusions about the nature and size of the mismatches between the clinical case and relevant study(ies). The inferred mismatches are used to compare treatment plans. Finally, the system's conclusions are passed to a text-generation program (described in Chapter 7) which assembles a prose critique.

Examples

Below are two examples of Roundsman using clinical studies to critique a physician's plan. The examples include a verbatim transcript of Roundsman's output. As mentioned earlier, to use Roundsman, physicians first describe their patient and propose a therapy choice. In these examples the physician has described a patient as follows: a 45 year-old pre-menopausal woman with a tumor size of 1.5 centimeters,

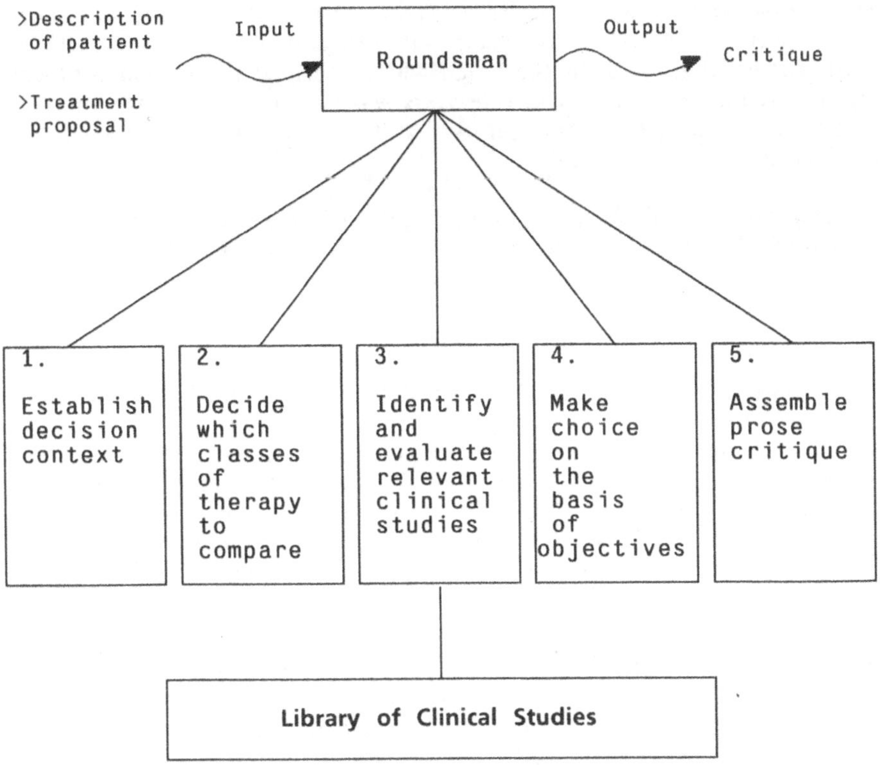

Figure 1-1: Flow of control in the Roundsman system.

clinically palpable axillary nodes (lymph nodes detected by physical exam) suspected of containing cancer, and no known metastases. The physician has also proposed a therapeutic plan of surgical wide excision followed by adjuvant radiotherapy (radiotherapy added to a surgical procedure).

Roundsman then produces a prose critique of this plan. In these introductory examples Roundsman critiques each relevant study serially without commenting upon the overall impact of a group of studies. The following verbatim transcript first shows Roundsman discussing the relevance of a publication by Peters [Peters 77]:

> "There are 2 studies pertinent to this patient.
>
> "First, Peters77 employed non-randomized controls in a study performed by investigators at Princess Margaret Hospital, Toronto. A set of patients who were treated by wide excision combined with adjuvant radiotherapy (N=203) is compared against treatment with radical mastectomy combined with adjuvant radiotherapy (N=609). For patients who underwent the first protocol the recurrence-free survival at five

years turned out to be 0.7, recurrence-free survival at ten years was equal to 0.6, overall survival at five years was 0.85 and overall survival at ten years was equal to 0.75. In the group which received the second protocol the recurrence-free survival at five years was 0.7, recurrence-free survival at ten years was 0.6, overall survival at five years was 0.8 and overall survival at ten years was 0.68.

"How do these data apply to your patient? We are not particularly concerned that the intervention was somewhat nonstandard (about 10% of each group didn't get the radiotherapy). More troublesome is that the study population was probably in a better prognostic stratum than your patient (they were clinically node negative).

"Reviewing the study itself, the results are weakened because first, statistical reporting was sketchy (data reported as graphs without P values or standard errors). Second, we suspect that a selection bias was introduced (e.g., tumor size assessed by same physicians who chose treatment). Third, choice of treatment was decided non-randomly (although Peters did match controls for T size, age & treatment year). Fourth, patients were accrued over a rather long period (patient entry lasted from 1939 to 1972). "

The critique begins by identifying the site of the investigation, specifying what treatments were compared, and reporting the outcomes which were observed. The second paragraph discusses how well the study generalizes to the particular patient and proposed treatment. The last paragraph critiques the study's methodology.

The second of the two studies cited by Roundsman for this patient and plan is a publication by Atkins [Atkins 72]:

" Second, Atkins72 was a randomized, controlled trial carried out at Guy's Hospital, England. Patients were randomized to wide excision combined with adjuvant radiotherapy (N=70) or to treatment with radical mastectomy combined with adjuvant radiotherapy (N=80). In the group which received the first protocol the proportion free of local or regional recurrence at five years was equal to 0.52 and overall survival at five years turned out to be 0.56. In the group which received the second protocol the proportion free of local or regional recurrence at five years turned out to be 0.84 and overall survival at five years was equal to 0.72.

"Are these results relevant to your patient? It is encouraging that your patient fits the study population extremely well (it was a clinical stage II population). We suspect it makes little difference that the study protocol included a modality beyond your proposed treatment (from 1961-68 both groups got small doses of Thiotepa, but this was shown to be ineffectual so it was discontinued), or that your patient's menopausal status is different (study subjects were post-menopausal, but since chemotherapy wasn't used this difference might be ignored). More troublesome is that their therapy was suboptimal (2500 rads of radiation is too low by today's standards).

"Judging the study as a biomedical report, among the strong points we note that controls were randomly assigned. The results are weakened because statistical reporting was sketchy (standard errors are not given)."

To further illustrate how Roundsman tailors its critique, the final transcript (below) shows how a different patient might cause Roundsman to direct its analysis to a different stratum in a study's population. Whereas in the earlier critique of Atkins72 the size of the two relevant study groups was 70 and 80 (see the first paragraph of the Atkins critique above), these sizes and the observed outcome fractions all change when the patient is stage I rather than stage II:

"Atkins72 was a randomized, controlled trial performed by investigators at Guy's Hospital, England. Subjects were assigned to wide excision combined with adjuvant radiotherapy (N=112) or another protocol which was radical mastectomy combined with adjuvant radiotherapy (N=108). For patients who underwent the first protocol the the proportion free of local or regional recurrence at five years was equal to 0.8 and overall survival at five years turned out to be 0.78. Under the second protocol the proportion free of local or regional recurrence at five years was 0.92 and overall survival at five years turned out to be 0.8."

These changes follow from the selection of a different patient population stratum on which to base the critique. The system can also react to a different treatment proposal. If, for example, the user's proposed therapy differed from the example given above, it is possible that neither Peters77 nor Atkins72 would enter into the critique at all.

As can be seen from these examples, a useful assessment of these publications goes far beyond mere reporting of statistical results. These critiques exhibit more fundamental knowledge of the experiment, bringing expert clinical judgment into the analysis.

1.4. Research Contributions

The research contribution of the Roundsman project can best be understood by viewing Roundsman from the perspectives of artificial intelligence, medical decision analysis, and bibliographic retrieval. (These fields are discussed in more detail in Chapter 2.)

The techniques of *artificial intelligence* are being applied to an increasing variety of problems. Biomedicine and the social sciences will repeatedly present problem domains for which there are no reliable causal models. In those domains, system designers might retreat to the surface-level heuristics which sufficed for first-generation expert systems. Instead, we suggest the investigation of how experts reason from the relevant bodies of experimental evidence. This evidence may well have its own structure (as is the case for clinical literature) which is tremendously useful when combined with knowledge about how to reason based on this structure. Building computer-based models of this reasoning process may yield useful decision support systems and may also illuminate general principles of reasoning from experimental evidence, opening these principles up to further explicit analysis.

One of the most difficult and time-consuming parts of performing medical *decision analysis* is estimating the probability of events. It is a task which requires a strong clinical background and experience reading biostatistical reports. Furthermore, this task is common to a variety of methodological approaches, from standard decision trees to Markov processes. There has been little explicit analysis, however, of the reasoning process by which probabilities are assigned, and (to our knowledge) no attempts to model it in a computer-based advice system. The Roundsman project explores the underlying reasoning process involved in making these assessments.

Unlike many current computer-based medical advice programs, *bibliographic retrieval* systems often meet immediate enthusiasm by clinicians. In these systems full-text copies (or abstracts) of journal articles are retrieved by a keyword index, which may be organized in a disease hierarchy, or according to the keyword's proximity to another keyword. These journal articles have the potential to change management decisions [Scura 81]. The state of this science however, is quite primitive: Matching strings of alphanumeric characters falls far short of "intelligent" information retrieval. The current Roundsman system is a step toward the development of systems which understand the structure of the literature they are searching, and can make inferences about how an article might relate to the clinical problem which a physician faces.

1.5. Guide to the Reader

Chapter 2 provides the backround which readers may require to understand the book.

Chapter 3 is a global overview of the Roundsman project and the Roundsman computer program which is its central focus. Section 3.1 describes how the model of reasoning from the clinical literature emerged from informal protocol analysis with an expert oncologist. Section 3.2 describes the development of a set of "scripts":

fictional critiques of a physician's proposed plan to manage a particular patient with primary breast cancer. These scripts served as targets during program development and they also helped to identify the set of publications which were incorporated into the Roundsman library (as described in section 3.3). Section 3.4 lists the hardware and software support used in program development. Section 3.5 outlines the steps taken by Roundsman when analyzing a case and then describes each of those steps in detail by tracing the execution of the system during an actual consultation.

Chapter 4 describes an open-ended distance metric designed to help assess the relevance of a study to a particular decision. It is open-ended in the sense that the passage of time may introduce *new* components into the metric (e.g., as new issues of interpretation are identified). It captures the *semantics* of the mismatch between study and clinical decision i.e., nuances that are key to producing a useful critique. Although a numeric (probabilistic) distance measure is included, the goal of the system is first and foremost to provide the user with contextual details of the mismatch rather than a mere assessment of its relative magnitude. The physician is then able to use his judgment in interpreting any distances as they apply to the patient. The distance metric has three purposes: (1) characterizing mismatches, (2) measuring mismatches and (3) helping correct for mismatches.

Chapter 5 explores a model of choice and explanation in medical management and makes clear its advantages and limitations. The model is based on multiattribute decision making and consists of four distinct strategies for choice and explanation, plus combinations of these four. The use of the strategies for both choice and explanation are illustrated with examples from the management of primary breast cancer, and also with reviews of several existing medical management AI systems. (The model lets us better understand and characterize the seemingly ad hoc decision making of these previous systems.) A simplified implementation of the model in Roundsman is described in this chapter. This approach to choice and explanation is independent of Roundsman's model of the clinical literature. Roundsman's knowledge representation for clinical studies and the use of the distance metric would be equally valid for a different approach to choice and explanation.

Chapter 6 discusses several settings in which interactions between studies play a prominent role in reasoning from the literature. One such setting is when newly published studies affect the interpretation of prior publications. A second situation in which inter-study relationships become central to problem-solving is when experimental results are in conflict. In the current Roundsman system, there is no representation of inter-study relationships. Although Roundsman does not currently deal with such interactions, I have devoted this chapter to setting down my current thoughts on the subject in an organized fashion. Thus, this chapter provides a preliminary skeleton upon which future research can build.

Chapter 7 describes the design of Roundsman's text generation subprogram. This chapter describes the required data structures in terms generic to object-oriented programming. The purpose of the chapter is to make clear exactly what is required to build and use this text-generation approach in *any* object-oriented programming language.

Chapter 8 provides extended examples of the Roundsman system in operation, and discusses additional system features. This chapter also discusses an evaluation of the Roundsman system.

Chapter 9 summarizes the principal research contributions, discusses limitations of the Roundsman project, and suggests promising areas for future research.

Chapter 2
Background

This chapter reviews the literature of several fields that relate to the subject of this book. Since readers will have varying backgrounds, some sections may be more familiar than others.

Section 2.1 reviews the field of artificial intelligence in medicine. The next three sections contrast Roundsman with consultation systems for biostatistics (2.2), computer databases (2.3), and computer programs for decision analysis (2.4). Section 2.5 discusses the classification of biomedical reports and identifies the type of study contained in Roundsman's library. Section 2.6 reviews written guides to the clinical application of biomedical reports. Section 2.7 defines medical terms which are necessary to understand the examples in this book.

2.1. A Review of Artificial Intelligence in Medicine

2.1.1. Introduction

For several decades, collaborating computer scientists and physicians have been building computer programs to diagnose medical illness and to recommend therapy. In the early 1970's, four research groups developed programs which differed somewhat from the other medical decision making programs in that they drew heavily on earlier artificial intelligence (AI) research such as DENDRAL, a program from the late 1960's that had used expert knowledge to derive chemical structure from mass spectral data [Buchanan 78]. The resulting work helped define the field of Artificial Intelligence in Medicine (AIM), and seeded development of expert systems in other domains as well [Szolovits 83, Clancey 84a].

Domains of both medical diagnosis and patient management helped demonstrate the validity of an emerging AI principle: that extensive domain-specific *knowledge* about a problem area are generally more crucial to problem-solving performance than are domain-independent *principles of reasoning*. In other words, simple reasoning techniques were shown to suffice for expert level performance so long as the program had comprehensive and accurate knowledge of the domain.

AIM research activities are important to medicine not only because medical advice systems will someday become routine tools in clinical practice, but also because the education of doctors, which has traditionally emphasized memorization of knowledge, may increasingly emphasize the learning of effective problem solving techniques, enhanced with the knowledge and advice provided by computer systems.

2.1.2. Theoretical Basis

Protocol Analysis

The theoretical foundation of AIM owes a great deal to psychological research that was carried out in the mid-1970's. In these experiments, physicians were urged to verbalize their thoughts while solving diagnostic problems. Researchers then analyzed transcripts of those sessions. Investigations of this type [Kassirer 78, Elstein 78] identified a general problem-solving procedure common to both expert and novice physicians: the hypothetico-deductive approach. Hypotheses emerge quite soon after the physician begins gathering data, and these are tested as new data arrives. Questions may be generated solely to test an active hypothesis, or to distinguish between hypotheses. Thus, early generation of hypotheses seems to provide leverage for the diagnostician.

Building on those results, researchers at the University of Minnesota [Feltovich 80] examined the performance of both experts and novices, and found differences not in their reasoning -- regardless of experience, they shared the hypothetico-deductive approach -- but in the richness and organization of medical knowledge. Novices had spotty knowledge of diesases, not yet full enough or sufficiently organized to optimize the hypothetico-deductive approach. These results agreed with the results of the expert systems research mentioned earlier, in that performance seemed to be critically dependent on domain-specific knowledge, rather than on sophisticated mechanisms for manipulating that knowledge.

Knowledge Representation

Two aspects of knowledge representation are of particular interest in considering the construction of medical advice systems. First, what knowledge do physicians use to make the diagnosis and to plan therapy? Second, what abstract data types are best for computer implementations of that knowledge? It became increasingly clear that the first-generation AIM programs captured only a small portion of the knowledge that physicians actually use in problem solving.

Typically, the medical knowledge represented in early systems consisted of weighted associations between findings (i.e., observable descriptors of a patient) and hypotheses, or between two hypotheses. The underlying semantics of such associations were not always made clear, and there was generally no distinction made between causal and associational relationships. For example, a diagnostic system might represent a link between the hypothesis of breast cancer and the finding that the patient's mother had breast cancer. In this case the finding is a risk factor, not a clear causal relationship as a skiing accident might be to a fractured leg.

In recent years AIM research has explored various representations for causal knowledge, and their integration into advice systems. Pure causal modelling, however, is rarely applicable in medicine because medicine is an empirical science in which detailed mechanisms are often unknown. Whenever cause-effect information *is* available to physicians, they can use it in at least five ways:

1. If one can confidently follow effect-to-cause links (i.e., statements of what entities may *cause* an observed effect) from the patient's complaints back toward primary disorders, an intersection point provides the diagnostician with a common cause of multiple complaints. CASNET is a computer program developed at Rutgers for the diagnosis and treatment of glaucoma; that domain lent itself to this intersection-point technique [Kulikowski 82, Weiss 78].

2. Medical therapy is often unavailable either for the patient's complaints or for the elemental physiologic disorder (primary disease) at the beginning of the causal path. But effective therapy may indeed be available for intermediate states. For example, swollen, painful feet can be caused by abnormal retention of fluid in the body, which is in turn caused by cardiomyopathy. Current medical therapy cannot correct cardiomyopathy, and it would be suboptimal to simply give pain killers for swollen feet, but drug therapy *can* reverse the fluid retention (intermediate state) and thus relieve the patient of swollen feet.

3. Physicians use causal models to interpret the temporal ordering of complaints. Leg cramps that occur during vigorous walking may be due to atherosclerotic disease, in which the leg muscles begin consuming more oxygen than the narrowed leg arteries can deliver. Leg cramps that are relieved by walking can not be explained by this mechanism.

4. Causal information can be used by a diagnostician to avoid treating two related findings as though they provide independent support for an hypothesis. For example, if there are known associations between findings f_j, f_k and hypothesis H, observation of both f_j and f_k might be interpreted as contributing independently to confidence in H. But if it is known that the causal path is $H \dashrightarrow f_j \dashrightarrow f_k$, then f_j and f_k must be dependent. Cooper [Cooper 84] uses causal models in this way to establish probability bounds which are consistent with knowledge about cause and effect.

5. Physicians use causal models to partition their knowledge into levels of abstraction. Diagnosis and explanation can then be performed at the clinical level (e.g., fatigue) or the pathophysiological level (e.g., serum partial pressure of carbon dioxide in blood is related algebraically to pH), depending upon the complexity of the problem and the demands for explanation. ABEL, a computer program developed at MIT to deal with acid-base and electrolyte disorders, first demonstrated the advantages of using such levels of abstraction [Patil 81].

Another area of increasing emphasis has been the representation of a taxonomy (i.e., hierarchic organization) for the diagnostic hypothesis space. For example, viral hepatitis and alcoholic hepatitis are both inflammatory diseases of the liver. A representation scheme that captures this type of hierarchic relationship might allow the system to begin reasoning at an appropriate level of abstraction, e.g., to identify a patient as having hepatitis before beginning to determine which subtype is present. Disease taxonomies, therefore, have been used to direct search. The MDX system, a liver disease diagnostic program developed at Ohio State University, contains a taxonomy of diseases which allows the system to direct the search as a progressive refinement of hypotheses, popping back to higher levels in the hierarchy only when strong inconsistencies arise [Gomez 81]. Another control scheme which uses taxonomic knowledge extensively can be found in the design for enhancements to INTERNIST, a diagnostic program for internal medicine developed at the University of Pittsburgh [Pople 82].

The abstract data types used in AIM systems have been legion, but three classes predominate: production rules, frames, and semantic networks. AIM researchers have not been uniform in their choice of knowledge representations. Four early AIM computer programs exemplified this diversity of representation schemes: MYCIN experimented with production rules; PIP and INTERNIST used disease frames; and CASNET represented causal relations in an associational network. An excellent discussion of knowledge representation in these four early AIM systems can be found in [Szolovits 78]. Support for the definition of abstract data types is provided by "object-centered programming" languages, which can be used to bind algorithms to the data structures on which they operate. Many computer scientists feel that the development of large systems is more manageable with this encapsulation scheme, and it still allows designs that use production rules, frames or networks. Several object-centered languages facilitate the construction of taxonomies by providing automatic inheritance of capabilities from object types to subtypes.

Control

Separation of the knowledge base (data structures) and control (algorithms) is often cited as a central element in expert system design and is a goal of most AIM system designers since this preserves the ability to work with each component separately. Designers can experiment with new control schemes, keeping the knowledge base fixed, and observe performance changes. For example, a new technique for combining evidence might be run on the MYCIN knowledge base, a collection of rules for making infectious disease diagnoses. Or a new INTERNIST-derived differential diagnosis mode might be run on the otherwise unaltered knowledge base. Also, knowledge acquisition, a primary concern of medical advice systems, can ideally be achieved by adding new instantiations of a data structure (e.g., a new rule or a new disease frame), thereby upgrading the knowledge base without changing the control structure.

There are as many control schemes as there are systems, and a large number of terms in use to describe control:

- MYCIN uses a backward-chaining depth-first control strategy to invoke and link its rules so that a reasoning network is created dynamically.
- INTERNIST's control is initially a data-directed scheme but evolves into an hypothesis-directed approach after an initial set of hypotheses is established [Miller, R. A. 82].
- The Serum Protein Diagnostic Program, built with an expert system building tool known as EXPERT [Weiss 81] does not require hypothesis-directed control because question selection is not a problem; most of the information is obtained automatically from an electrophoresis instrument with which this program is packaged and sold. Thus its control is predominantly data-directed.
- The control strategy of Ohio State's MDX system [Gomez 81] is a breadth-first search of a static tree. As MDX pushes deeper into this taxonomy tree, it is refining hypotheses to be more specific.
- The ATTENDING system, developed at Yale to critique anesthesia management plans [Miller 83a, Miller 84], searches a hierarchical planning network in order to identify alternatives to the user's proposed plan. Starting at the most detailed arcs of this augmented transition network, ATTENDING compares the risks of the user's proposed arc (action) to the risks of parallel arcs.

Evaluation Functions

AI chess playing programs use an evaluation function to assign numeric values to board positions. Advice systems in medical management face analogous situations, but the values of medical outcomes can be very difficult to assess. What are the relative values of chronic pain versus a lifetime of paralysis versus loss of life? The absence of a generally accepted "correct" therapy means that the physician will demand a reasoned argument which addresses the issues of costs and benefits in a convincing way. This issue is of growing importance to medical AI researchers because there is increasing interest in designing therapy systems.

Diagnosis systems typically sidestep the difficulties of evaluation functions, except as they relate to test selection during a diagnostic workup. Most of these systems consider information-gathering costs, but this does not constitute a comprehensive value theory for medical advice systems because it ignores the utility of acts, i.e., the cost of incorrect action. For example, assume that a medical advice system concludes that an infection is most likely caused by organism-1, and much less likely by organism-2. Is it correct management to treat for organism-1 and not for organism-2? Perhaps not if organism-1 causes only discomfort while organism-2 can cause death and the treatment for organism-1 may cause kidney damage. The cost of diagnostic misclassification drives the real-life diagnostic process. Medical cost containment pressures may force more explicit inclusion of cost/benefit considerations in decision support systems as well. Future research is likely to draw upon related disciplines such as operations research which provide a formal theory for evaluating the expected utility of actions.

Inexact Inference (for scoring hypotheses)

"Inexact inference" in this discussion refers to use of information which is probabilistic to some degree, rather than purely categorical. Medical evidence is such that most conclusions can be drawn only with a limited degree of certainty. This character of medical evidence and hypothesis assessment has driven AIM researchers to experiment with different scoring schemes. Few AIM systems have used classical probability theory to represent uncertainty. Systems developed in medical centers have tended to seek representations for uncertainty which reflect physician behavior, and several researchers have argued that probability theory and the use of Bayes' Theorem do not model that behavior well [Shortliffe 75]. They further argued that the application of Bayes' theorem often requires so many simplifying assumptions that the theoretical foundations tend to be invalidated in any practical system using a probabilistic approach. Thus, more ad hoc approaches have become competitors for representation of uncertainty.

The MYCIN experiments resulted in the certainty factor model [Shortliffe 75]. The INTERNIST project produced a calculus of evoking strength and frequency weights [Miller, R. A. 82]. These alternatives vary in their degree of formalism. It is expected that future work will better elucidate the features of these alternatives which were not seen in probability theory. On the other hand, the perceived differences between formal systems like probability theory and the alternatives may diminish as researchers identify how the advantages of each can be melded in medical advice systems.

2.1.3. Research Themes

Additional ongoing research topics for investigators building AIM systems for diagnosis or management advice include the following:

Knowledge Acquisition

A well-recognized bottleneck in building expert systems is acquiring knowledge from the expert. Work on TEIRESIAS, a program built to interface with MYCIN [Davis 79], demonstrated that a program might assist in the on-line transfer of knowledge from a human expert to the consultation program's knowledge base. If the expert disagrees with a conclusion, the system traces, step-by-step, back through the reasoning process until an erroneous rule (or missing rule) is identified. The SEEK program, which operates in concert with the EXPERT program mentioned earlier, also provides assistance in recognizing how a system's knowledge base should be altered [Politakis 82]. Focussing on actual cases, the system suggests refinements to the knowledge base, which take the form of adding or deleting the number of "major findings" or "minor findings" of a disease needed to satisfy a diagnostic rule.

Explanation

MYCIN was one of the first systems to demonstrate that explanation capabilities might be key to physician acceptance of computer-based decision support [Scott 77]. MYCIN allowed users to ask "why?", when they were unclear about the purpose of the system's questioning, and "how?" when they wanted to know how the system would (or did) reach certain conclusions. Researchers at MIT enriched the Digitalis Therapy Advisor [Gorry 78] with causal models of heart rhythm disturbances, and principles of anti-arrhythmia therapy to create a computer program named XPLAIN [Swartout 81] which could give the rationale behind a therapy.

This work demonstrated that optimal explanation was facilitated by access to the more abstract principles which do not always appear in the program code. In a similar spirit, the goals of the NEOMYCIN project at Stanford University are to provide explanation of the diagnostic process in terms of diseases and symptoms but also in terms of the over-arching principles of medical diagnosis. This work has included a revision of MYCIN's rules and the addition of an explicit model of diagnostic strategy [Hasling 84, Clancey 81].

The ATTENDING system for anesthesia management planning first proposed a critiquing approach to explanation [Miller 83a, Miller 84]. Rather than simulating a physician's reasoning and generating a recommended action, critiquing systems center their analysis around the user's proposed management plan. In medical management there is often more than one defensible therapy, so an approach that highlights the pros and cons of each approach is more likely to meet acceptance by the physician. In addition, critiquing systems remain silent on the uncontroversial aspects of the plan.

Temporal reasoning

Medical advice systems are usually designed with the assumption that data are gathered and inferences are made at one point in time. Since medical diagnosis and management actually take place over time, optimal medical advice systems will allow 1) reevaluation of the patient, 2) assessing the rate of disease progression or 3) assessing the therapeutic response to prior treatment. The Digitalis Therapy Advisor, VM and ONCOCIN are unusual in that they have attempted to manage patients over time. The Digitalis Therapy Advisor [Gorry 78] uses the results of previous treatment to alter its model of the patient. For example, if predicted body stores of digitalis are much higher than measured stores, then the system adjusts the "oral absorption" parameter downwards. VM, a program designed to assist with the management of patients on respiratory support systems (mechanical ventilators), assumes that particular data are only valid for a certain period of time, and the system can represent temporal trends [Fagan 79]. An example of this is VM's ability to detect a rise in mean arterial blood pressure of 15 torr over 10 minutes. ONCOCIN [Shortliffe 81] follows patients through many cycles of cancer chemotherapy, each cycle lasting weeks. Some of its inference rules test temporal trends of patient parameters.

Validation

Diagnosis systems are usually judged by the accuracy of their diagnosis when compared to some accepted "gold standard". Credibility is gained by evaluating the program, informally at first and then in double-blinded studies. Several groups have carried out formal evaluations of performance [Yu 79, Miller, R. A. 82, Aikins 83, Hickam 85].

Evaluation in a different clinical setting from that in which the system was built can help to demonstrate generalizability. Fewer groups have evaluated the acceptability to users. Indeed, success in this area is notoriously difficult to achieve. Systems that involve hands-on use by doctors face additional challenging design issues compared to those systems which analyze instrument data and produce a report. Objectives and guidelines for system validation are discussed in Chap. 30 of [Buchanan 84].

Designing for Clinical Use

The CASNET research at Rutgers led to the first commercial application of AI in medicine, the Serum Protein Diagnostic Program [Weiss 81]. Two other AIM systems in clinical use are PUFF [Aikins 83], and ONCOCIN [Shortliffe 81]. All three of these systems are used by practicing doctors. The design requirements of PUFF and the Serum Protein Diagnostic Program are quite different from that of ONCOCIN however. Both of those systems acquire the needed information automatically from instruments, so that data collection, analysis and recommendation can proceed without direct interaction with the physician. This is quite different from ONCOCIN, where the physician's hands-on interaction with the computer is a major design consideration. In general, systems that will be used interactively face additional design challenges: response-time must be short, data collection and analysis must be simple and intuitive to the physician, recommendations must be backed up with good explanations, and finally system hardware and software must be reliably available.

2.1.4. Summary of Roundsman's Relationship to Prior AIM Research

As described in section 2.1.2, the medical knowledge of early AIM systems often consisted of weighted associations between findings and hypotheses, or between two hypotheses. These links represented the "distilled" heuristics of practicing physicians. As experience with these systems grew, it became increasingly clear that effective problem-solving of difficult cases requires additional knowledge: more fundamental models ("deep knowledge") of the problem domain. (A similar need was perceived by researchers in computer-aided instruction [Sleeman 81].) There was a strong sense in the AIM community during the early 1980's that the research frontier was (a) elucidating the nature of these models and (b) finding knowledge representations that could allow a machine to make use of this information.

Subsequent research efforts have concentrated on *causal models*, most notably the research of Patil on ABEL [Patil 81]. This research combines detailed physiological models of the human body with surface-level heuristics (which the first generation of AIM systems had used). This causal modeling direction is reinforced by simultaneous work in modeling electronic circuits in order to build expert systems to help debug computer hardware. Indeed, there is lively discussion in the AIM field of whether *qualitative* causal models can serve in lieu of more quantitative causal models, but there has been little discussion of the limitations that the causal model paradigm might have for modeling expert reasoning.

The Roundsman project is modeling a type of fundamental knowledge that is quite different from causal models. Rapidly-changing technical fields (e.g., medical management) present problems for which detailed causal models do not yet exist. As mentioned in section 2.1.2, medicine is an empirical science in which pathophysiologic mechanisms are often unknown. In these situations the clinician's reasoning is based upon experimental evidence from clinical studies reported in the medical literature. The research described in this book, and the Roundsman computer program, are a first step toward modeling that process of reasoning from experimental evidence.

In addition to providing an alternative approach to *causal modeling*, the Roundsman project builds upon prior AIM research in several other ways. Informal *protocol analysis* with the collaborating oncologist (described in Chapter 3) provides the rough model of how the oncologist reasons from the clinical literature. The design of Roundsman's *evaluation function* (described in Chapter 5) draws upon an operations research perspective of prior AIM systems. The importance of system *explanation* capabilities, made abundantly clear by research in AIM, is the impetus for our efforts to generate text from Roundsman (discussed in Chapter 7). The major departure from previous research is the proposition that AIM research will greatly strengthen its clinical utility if it broadens its research focus beyond causal modeling and examines reasoning from experimental evidence reported in the clinical literature.

2.2. Consultation Systems for Biostatistics

This section outlines several ways in which consultation systems might assist biostatistical analysis and describes several research projects to build such systems. In general, the biostatistical systems described in this section are less clinically oriented than the AIM systems described in section 2.1.

The broad range of biostatistical activities in medicine suggests several ways in which biostatistical consultation systems might be useful:

- Exploratory data analysis: Biostatisticians often review patient data in an exploratory manner in order to discover associations or trends which are not anticipated in advance. A large patient data base may suggest a number of interesting hypotheses. Confirmation of these hypotheses requires a planned experiment. (A certain number of apparent associations between data will occur by chance alone. Clearly, the potential for finding false-positive associations is quite high when one is essentially "fishing" for relationships in the data.)

- Planning experiments: Biomedical researchers often do not know exactly what experimental design will best answer the principal research question(s). Poor planning makes the experimental results - obtained at the cost of time, money and effort - much less valuable for statistical inference. One reason that biostatisticians are in great demand at centers of medical research it that they provide advice on experimental design. A consultation system which could effectively assist with this task would also be in great demand.

- Advise users of computer-based statistical packages: Computer software has broadened the audience that can perform statistical analyses. Unfortunately, this increases the chance that statistical techniques will be applied to problems for which they are not suited. To perform effective statistical analysis it is necessary to understand the assumptions underlying statistical techniques and also to understand the domain of application well enough to judge whether those assumptions are reasonable.

- Evaluate the statistical methodology of biomedical reports: The quality of a biomedical report is dependent upon factors such as the sample size, the method of control (e.g., randomization), the completeness of follow-up, and similar issues in the statistical design. Weakness in any of several methodological design issues can undermine the validity of the experimental results.

Several statistical consultation systems address some of the challenges mentioned above. For example, the goals of the RX project at Stanford [Blum 82] are to generate and test hypotheses by examining a medical database. Hypotheses that withstand testing might then become the basis for inclusion in the system's knowledge base. The system consists of several modules: the *discovery module* detects associations in the data base which suggest causal relationships in the form of "A causes B", the *study module* develops a statistical model designed to test the hypothesis, and the *statistical analysis module* tests the hypothesis. The study module (the most well developed of the three modules) uses stored knowledge of confounding relationships to develop a test for a proposed causal hypothesis.

The GUHA-80 project in Czechoslovakia [Hajek 82] has aims which are similar to those of the RX project. They seek to emphasize the automatic formation of hypotheses: the program is designed to develop interesting views of empirical data. Statistical analysis of those views is not the primary research emphasis, although there are plans to include a statistical package as well.

There is little reported research on systems designed to help plan the statistical design of experiments. One preliminary report concerns a program named

EXPERIPLAN [Schreiner 84]. The purpose of that program is to help users design statistical experiments in order to test complex hypotheses. This research is not yet developed enough to provide a detailed description of its design, but it serves as another example of an application of consultation systems to biostatistics.

As mentioned earlier in this section, there are computer programs available to perform complex statistical analysis, but these require significant statistical expertise to use the program correctly. A research team at AT&T Bell Laboratories is designing a regression expert system to help novice users perform regression analysis on data [Gale 82]. This program, named REX, detects and corrects violations of assumptions made by standard regression techniques. If the program finds that the assumptions are not met it may suggest changes to the data or to the model. A feasibility demonstration has been constructed in which statistical knowledge is represented in frames. REX complement the RX system (mentioned earlier) because REX is not capable of automatically designing tests and RX does not emphasize the checking of a model's assumptions before testing.

The goal of the REFEREE [Haggarty 84] program is to assist in the initial evaluation of a clinical study's statistical methodology. The system asks its user (e.g., a journal referee) about the sample size, whether the experiment was blind, what percentage of patients were followed up, and so on. The end result is an integer score which represents the system's assessment of the study's (methodological) "validity".

Since Roundsman and REFEREE both concern clinical studies, it is useful to understand how the two projects differ and also how they complement each other. Roundsman critiques a specific therapy proposal for a particular patient with primary breast cancer. The REFEREE program does not address a particular clinical management decision, it's advice is not specific to a patient, and the system is not knowledgeable about a medical domain. The purposes of the two programs are therefore quite different. Along one dimension however, the design goals of REFEREE and Roundsman complement each other nicely: REFEREE might identify methodological weaknesses by questioning the user about the study's methodological approach. It might then store judgments about methodology (rather than producing an integer score) which Roundsman could use later. However, issues of interpretation related to the specific patient and treatment proposal (not addressed by REFEREE) are key issues in Roundsman. There has been (to my knowledge) no previous research into the design of computer programs to assist in the *clinical* and *patient-specific* interpretation of the clinical trials literature.

This section is not exhaustive and there are worthwhile research projects which have not been mentioned. I have instead described a range of potential applications for consultation systems, and pointed out that the existing systems are, in general, much less clinically oriented than the AIM systems of section 2.1.

2.3. Computer Databases

2.3.1. Bibliographic Retrieval Systems

With the development of MEDLINE, the National Library of Medicine (NLM) pioneered research into bibliographic retrieval. This work certainly demonstrated that research physicians could utilize computer-based assistance in searching the medical literature. Interest in this and subsequent systems such as BRS, DIALOG, and Paperchase [Horowitz 81] suggests that *practicing* clinicians recognize a similar need [Doszkocs 80]. Indeed, Scura demonstrated that the assistance of a clinical librarian to identify case-specific literature could effectively change management decisions [Scura 81].

In certain respects, Roundsman's internal structures resemble a bibliographic retrieval system more than they resemble a traditional expert system. For example, information resides in separately identifiable "articles" rather than being merged into a knowledge base of clinical rules. Indeed, Roundsman is an exciting direction for research in bibliographic retrieval; yet as will be shown below, there are large differences between the Roundsman system and *current* bibliographic retrieval.

Literature database systems typically search for a user-specified sequence of alphanumeric characters. The machine understands very little of the medical domain. At most, a disease hierarchy might assist search (e.g., MEDLINE), but often only the proximity of one term to another guides the search (e.g., BRS). Thus the content and meaning of articles within a bibliographic retrieval system is inaccessible to the computer itself.

Researchers at the NLM have explored more concept-oriented approaches to storing information. Two such projects are the Hepatitis Knowledge Base experiment [Bernstein 80], and a similar project applied to human genetics (see Cummings, Chap. 10 in [Warren 81]). The Roundsman project differs from the Hepatitis Knowledge Base (KB) experiment in at least three ways:

1. The information in the Hepatitis KB is text (i.e., clusters of alphanumeric strings) augmented with a sophisticated index. In Roundsman, information is represented as data structures which are much more complex than text strings. Conclusions are drawn based on these data structures. Text strings are used only to communicate the conclusions to the physician and to insert connecting clauses into Roundsman's critique.

2. The Hepatitis KB includes any scientific information concerning hepatitis. For example, it includes descriptive information about the protein coat structure of the hepatitis virus. Roundsman is designed to represent clinical studies (solely). This is not a necessary restriction, but clarifies the current focus of the Roundsman project.

3. Roundsman *critiques* the literature (not simply retrieving it) in light of a *particular patient* and *specific treatment decision*. This is outside the scope of the Hepatitis KB experiment.

Ideally, it would be advantageous if Roundsman would scan the full-text article and interpret the information for itself and thereby eliminate the need for an expert oncologist to read and interpret the article.

There exist some programs capable of processing medical text, most notably those developed by the Linguistic String Project at NYU [Sager 78, Hirschman 81]. Those programs, however, use the somewhat restricted vocabulary and the stylized format of medical discharge summaries. Another research project, at SRI International, was specifically aimed at natural language understanding of the Hepatitis Knowledge Base [Walker 81]. But this natural language work is not yet mature enough for practical application. For an introductory review of text understanding systems, see [Sager 87].

2.3.2. Databases of Patient Records

A medical record contains information on the patient's medical history. A collection of computer-based medical records is often referred to as a "patient database". A patient database may have multiple uses: 1) physicians may use it in patient care, 2) administrators use it for billing, 3) researchers may use it for epidemiologic and biostatistical research, and 4) third-party payers may use it for reimbursement. In general, a patient database can adequately serve a particular purpose best if that use of the data was anticipated before collection of the data.

There is a great difference between Roundsman's knowledge base and patient databases. Publications of clinical studies do not report data at the level of individual patients, but rather for a "stratum" of patients. The stratum results are not a collection of individual patient records as would be found in a patient database. A stratum is a summary description for a portion of the study's population grouped together because of certain common characteristics such as age, sex, or disease type.

Clinical studies are *derived from* patient data which comprise, in the strictest sense, a "patient database". However, the conventional understanding of patient database more often means a set of data that was not collected as part of a study. Indeed, many difficulties in interpreting patient database information stem from the fact that the data are often entered without knowing precisely how they will used. In contrast, the most difficult (and crucial) part of carrying out a clinical study is assuring the integrity of the data that will be entered. Physician collaborators must be in close communication and the protocols must be carefully specified to avoid confounding variables as much as possible. Actual analysis of the data, once they are in a "database", is in many ways the easy part.

Furthermore, the "eligibility criteria" for entry of a patient into a patient database are often not well specified. Also, aggressive follow-up of patients is often not a primary goal. Finally, crisp definition of outcomes is not always present because there may be many diverse physicians making observations and entering data. If there is no standardization of terms (as one strives for in the course of a clinical study), the data may be very difficult to interpret.

Research in the use of databases of patient records has taken many directions, some of which have parallels with the Roundsman project. For example, there have been investigations into the use of specialty databases to yield prognostic information based on subsetting of the data [Rosati 75, deDombal 86]. This is in the same spirit as Roundsman because the researchers are looking for insight into individual patient prognoses.

Precisely because of the interpretation difficulties mentioned above, investigators have studied database designs which lend themselves to statistical research such as the explicit introduction of time [Weyl 75]. Building on the advantages introduced by a time-oriented schema, artificial intelligence researchers have looked at the potential for automatic hypothesis generation and testing [Blum 82]. Others have sought to tie the collection of patient data in with computer systems capable of clinical surveillance [Warner 72]. Although many patient data bases concern inpatients, it has been noted that an equally large potential for medical decision support exists with in database management systems for outpatient medical records [Barnett 84].

2.4. Decision Analysis

The discipline now known as medical decision analysis was virtually non-existent before a landmark paper by Ledley and Lusted characterized the science of medical practice as being composed of (a) probablistic reasoning, (b) value theory and (c) symbolic reasoning, and proposed that physicians examine their decision-making in terms of those three components [Ledley 59].

Articles using or discussing medical decision analysis now appear regularly in medical journals [Gorry 73, McNeil 75, Pauker 80, Pauker 81, McNeil 82]. The basic approach to decision analysis might be characterized as follows: (1) prepare a structure of a given clinical decision, for example a decision tree or Markov model, which represents the sequence of candidate decisions and chance outcomes, (2) assign probabilities to the various possible outcomes, (3) assign a utility value for each of the possible outcomes (4) weight the utilities by the probabilities to score the decisions, and (5) designate the decision with the best score as optimal. In addition, using techniques such as sensitivity analysis it is possible to determine the extent to which assumptions used in a formal model will affect the recommendation that is generated. This in turn helps determine whether further data and analysis are needed before a defensible decision can be reached.

Unfortunately, probabilities are rarely available for the clinical situation at hand. A critical reading of the clinical literature is often the source of these numbers. Case presentations and analysis in the journal *Medical Decision Making* invariably include statements about the literature reviewed and the interpretation of that literature [Moroff 83]. Nevertheless, there has been (to my knowledge) no attempt to build an explicit computational model of how physicians interpret the clinical literature in order to apply the results of biomedical reports to particular cases.

There is considerable interest among decision analysts in deciding whether the conclusions of studies are justified [Albert 81] and in formalizing ways in which published clinical studies can be "graded" [Begg 85]. This research is similar in spirit to the work by Chalmers (discussed below in Section 2.6) because it focusses on a report's biostatistical methodology rather than its relevance to a particular patient and specific decision. The DEALE model [Beck 82] suggests an approach to adjusting life expectancy estimates (these could be from a published study) to correct for coexisting diseases, as well as for age, sex and race. This model and it's relationship to Roundsman are discussed more fully in Chapter 4.

Currently, the computer programs which assist decision analysts do not help assess the clinical literature. Instead, the user typically constructs a decision tree and assigns probabilities which have *already* been assessed. The program calculates the expected value of each action being considered and helps perform sensitivity analysis on variables used in the model [Pauker 81, Doubilet 83]. Some preliminary research projects [Hollenberg 84] are examining how systems might possess enough domain knowledge to help the user select appropriate *branches* for the decision tree: suggesting additional branches or identifying branches of the current model which do not make sense. As mentioned earlier, the clinical literature is often the source for the probabilities used in this type of program. The process of assessing the clinical literature is outside the scope of these programs however. The goal of the Roundsman project is to implement a computational model of this process.

2.5. Scope of the Biomedical Reports in Roundsman's Library

Biomedical research reports can be classified along many dimensions, e.g., whether they use a randomized design or a non-randomized design, whether they are prospective or retrospective. Classification provides a framework to help understand the scope of the publications which are represented in Roundsman.

Within the classification scheme of [Bailar 84b], the breast cancer studies represented in Roundsman's knowledge base are longitudinal, prospective, studies of deliberate intervention (see Table 2-1). If computer-based representations of other classes were sought, somewhat different research issues would probably emerge. Cross-sectional studies differ from *longitudinal* studies in that longitudinal studies are particularly concerned with changes over time. For example, studies of the prevalence of heart disease in hypertensive people would be cross-sectional, whereas a study of the development of heart disease over a time period following intervention (to lower blood pressure) would be a longitudinal study.

Within longitudinal studies, there are *prospective* and *retrospective* studies. (Also known by the names *cohort* and *case-control*, respectively.) The key issue in distinguishing these two is whether the patients were selected for study on the basis of factors that are thought to influence outcome (prospective) or on the basis of endpoints being measured (retrospective). For example, if patients are selected and grouped according to whether they got a treatment for reducing high blood pressure, and are subsequently evaluated to determine their heart attack rate, it is a prospective study. If patients are selected because they had heart attacks, and then their use of the anti-hypertensive treatment is examined, it is a retrospective study. (It is irrelevant whether the events studied are to occur in the future, or have already occurred.)

Longitudinal prospective studies of deliberate intervention are further subclassified according to how experimental control is achieved (see Table 2-1). If the treatments are given to different patients in the same study, this is called *parallel control*. On the other hand, if the report compares (implicitly or explicitly) the results of treating study patients to patients outside the study (for example in another published study) then this is called *external control*. Parallel control and external control each occur in the literature on treatment of primary breast cancer. (Another design listed in Table 2-1, called sequential control, is not relevant to this literature.)

Many of Roundsman's studies use a parallel control design. Despite the tremendous advantages of this design, interpretation of the results is rarely straightforward [Lavori 83]. There are statistical questions: How stringent should the requirements be for "statistical significance"? If the difference between two treatments is *not* statistically significant, does this satisfactorily demonstrate that there is no

- Longitudinal studies
  - Prospective studies
    - Studies of deliberate intervention
      - Sequential
      - Parallel
      - External controls
    - Observational studies
      - Causes and incidence of disease
      - Deliberate but uncontrolled interventions
      - Natural history and prognosis
  - Retrospective studies
    - Studies of deliberate intervention
    - Observational studies
- Cross-sectional studies
  - Disease description
  - Diagnosis and staging
  - Disease processes

Table 2-1: Research report classification scheme from [Bailar 84b]. The studies known to Roundsman are longitudinal, prospective, studies of deliberate intervention.

difference? In addition, there are important *clinical* questions beyond these statistical questions: What patients were eligible for the study in the first place? (This bears on how a physician will view the applicability of the study to his particular patient.) The astute clinician will also want to know precisely what protocol (technique) was followed, to judge whether that technique is available to him in his practice, or is now considered out of date. Many of these *statistical* and *clinical* issues will be seen again in the chapters that follow.

The value of studies using external controls, and the difficulties of their interpretation, are addressed in [Moses 84] and also in [Bailar 84a]. Only a combination of both a clinical and a biostatistical perspective can provide a useful interpretation of this type of study. The difficulties of interpretation stem largely from the (usually) significant differences between patient groups being compared. There will be concern about whether the outcome differences truly reflect different treatment effects or just the differences between the patient groups. *There are no statistical adjustments that will automatically correct for these biases. Clinical judgments are required.* Nevertheless, most of medical practice has been derived from series-based information with no internal controls. The importance of externally-controlled studies is therefore apparent.

2.6. Guides to Clinical Application of Biomedical Reports

What has been written to help the clinician apply the results of clinical studies to individual patients? Very little, and what there is tends to be extremely cautious in its recommendations (wisely so, for this is a difficult area).

One of the best sources for this kind of advice is Biostatistics in Clinical Medicine [Ingelfinger 83]. Chapter 10 is entitled "Reading a Report of a Clinical Trial". This chapter attempts to provide some guidance for the critical reading of the clinical literature. In chapter 11, "Applying a Clinical Trial", the authors address the difficulties of using the study results to manage a specific patient. The authors do a superb job of explaining certain pitfalls, such as "fishing" for a subgroup with extreme results and then worrying about whether your patient fits those parameters rather than deciding *before* reading the report what clinical parameters are important. The guidelines provided are useful in a general way, but they require clinical expertise to be applied correctly. For example, in a section entitled "Comparing your patient to the study subjects", the authors advise:

> Check whether your patient would have been admitted to the study had it been held in your institution. If not, a good deal of judgment may be required. Your patient may have a different type of illness or therapy may be contraindicated. [Ingelfinger 83]

This leaves a good deal of room for subjective, clinical judgment. The authors go on to note that practicing physicians may not have available to them the precise therapeutic drugs or procedures that were used in a study, or may want to tailor a therapy somewhat differently from what was done in the study. This brings up the issue of changing a treatment protocol:

> If you, as a physician, modify a clinical trial protocol in applying the results to your patient, you assume that you have captured, in your modified therapy, that aspect of the protocol which caused the beneficial results. Although you and many other physicians may think the modifications reasonable, your modified therapy has not been tested and this adds uncertainty to the expected outcome. [ibid]

As can be seen from these excerpts, the advice is general. Indeed, without knowing the precise medical question being asked and the details of the study being examined, the most one can do is to offer general guidelines to the practicing physician.

Another useful book on this topic is Coping with the Biomedical Literature [Warren 81]. Chapter 9 is entitled "Evaluation: Requirements for Clinical Application". The author of that chapter, David Sackett, suggests performing a critical reading by asking directed questions such as "Were the study patients recognizably similar to your own?" and "Is the therapeutic maneuver replicable in your practice?" These are helpful, but very general guidelines. In other parts the author urges attention to methodology: "Were the patients randomized?", "Were there well-defined outcomes?", and "Was there complete follow-up of patients who entered the study?"

In a paper entitled "A method for assessing the quality of a randomized control trial", Chalmers focusses on statistical methodology [Chalmers 81]. He itemizes a checklist of items which might be used to assess the *methodological* quality of a randomized controlled trial. The author provides an explicit algorithm which others might use: the criteria for a successful "score" on each item are listed. There is no claim for a theoretical basis to the scoring: it is empirical, based on the expert opinion of biostatisticians.

Another source for guidelines to assessing biostatistical methodology is Statistics in Medicine [Colton 74], especially the chapter entitled "Critical Reading of the Medical Literature".

This section has described references which attempt to provide the practicing clinician with some tools to assess the applicability of a clinical study to his practice. The salient features of this type of advice are (1) that it is primarily biostatistical rather than clinical and (2) that it is general, requiring a significant refinement to tailor it to the clinical question at hand. Indeed, how could it be otherwise without knowledge of the problem domain? The job of applying these general "guidelines" in a particular clinical setting rests with the clinician. *As a result, Roundsman's knowledge about the studies in its knowledge base contains a significant amount of clinical judgment made by our domain expert.*

2.7. Management of Primary Breast Cancer

This section defines medical terms which are necessary to understand the examples found later in the book. The terms pertain to the management of primary breast cancer: treatment options, treatment objectives, and the therapeutic controversies.

2.7.1. Treatment Options

Management of primary breast cancer involves some combination of (a) surgery, (b) adjuvant radiotherapy, and (c) adjuvant systemic therapies such as hormonal therapy or chemotherapy. Our examples are limited to (a) and (b).

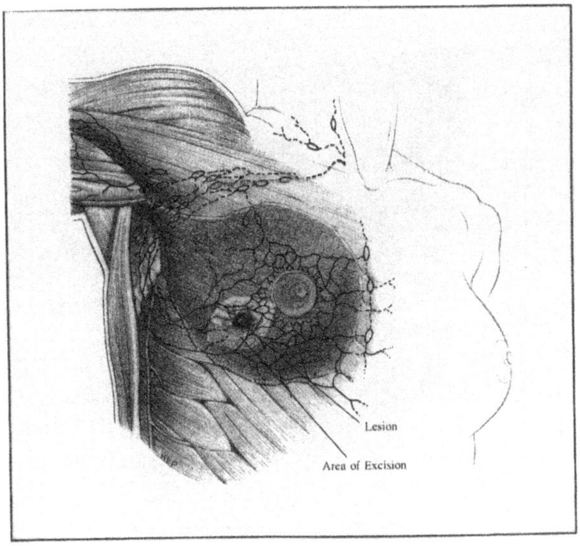

Figure 2-1: Local Excison.
The portion of the breast containing the tumor is surgically removed. Axillary lymph nodes may or may not be removed. (In this sketch they have not been removed). A *verified wide excision* is a local excision in which the margins of the excised tissue have been verified free of tumor. When a *quadrantectomy* is done, the surgeon removes the entire quadrant of the breast in which the tumor is located. Reprinted with permission from the journal *Resident and Staff Physician.*

Radical mastectomy: From the late 1800's until the 1970's, the most common surgical procedure for primary breast cancer was the radical mastectomy (see Fig. 2-3). The radical mastectomy (RM) leaves a severe cosmetic deformity of the chest wall because the chest wall musculature is removed in addition to the breast. This extensive removal of the muscles and lymphatic tissues adjacent to the tumor guarantees more complete removal of cancer tissue. Breast cancer, a lethal disease in a high proportion of women who acquire it, does not kill when localized to the breast: death results from the effect of metastatic deposits of cancer in *distant* parts of the body. Consequently, the central tenet of breast cancer therapy has been to surgically remove the cancer tissue before it could spread.

Total mastectomy: The most commonly used surgical procedure today is called a total mastectomy (TM). In this procedure all breast tissue is removed (see Fig. 2-2) but the pectoralis (chest wall) muscles remain intact. The surgeon may also dissect the axilla to remove the axillary lymph nodes. The choice between radical

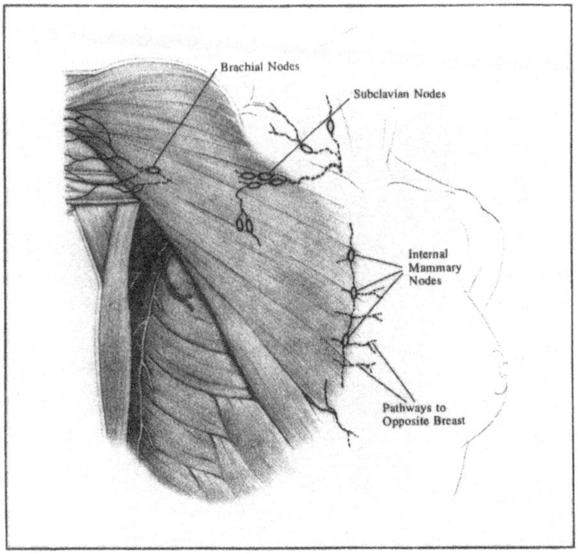

Figure 2-2: Total Mastectomy.

As in the radical mastectomy, the breast is removed. The chest wall muscles (pectoralis) however, are not removed. Axillary lymph nodes may or may not be removed. (In this sketch the axillary lymph nodes have been removed). Reprinted with permission from the journal *Resident and Staff Physician.*

mastectomy and total mastectomy was the subject of vehement debate for decades.

Wide excision: The controversial question today is whether total mastectomy might be replaced with wide excision (WE). Excision removes only the tumor, leaving as much breast tissue as possible (see Fig. 2-1). WE is advocated by some physicians even for patients in whom the tumor has reached the axillary lymph nodes. Consequently, this procedure directly violates a central tenet of cancer surgery: to achieve complete removal of cancer tissue if possible.

Adjuvant radiation therapy may follow the surgical procedure. (The adjective *adjuvant* indicates that the radiotherapy is used in combination with a surgical procedure.) Radiation is administered in daily treatments over a period of one or two weeks.

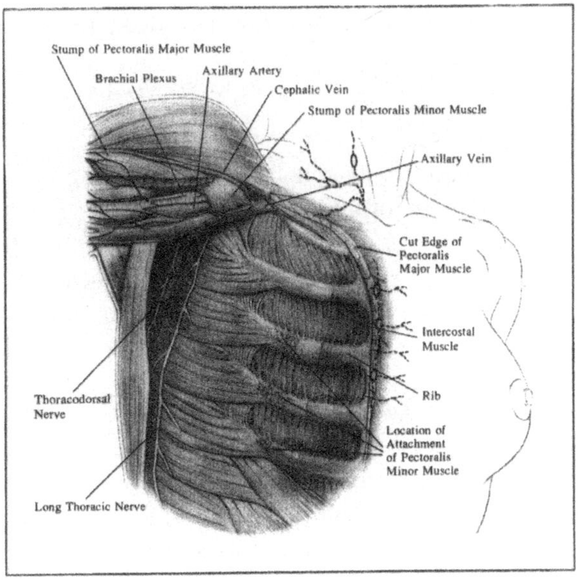

Figure 2-3: Halsted Radical Mastectomy.

This surgical procedure removes the breast, the pectoralis (chest wall) muscles and the axillary lymph nodes. Reprinted with permission from the journal *Resident and Staff Physician.*

2.7.2. Treatment Objectives

The medical management of a woman with primary breast cancer has several objectives. It is desirable to:

1. maximize the chance of cure
2. minimize the cosmetic damage of treatment
3. minimize the trauma of the procedure: hospital recovery time, repeated radiotherapy (RTX) visits, surgical morbidity, etc.
4. minimize the chance of tumor recurrence in the breast or chest wall even if the chance of overall survival is otherwise equivalent. (Relapse can occur in distant sites such as bone where the associated morbidity is usually less than that of relapse in the chest wall.)
5. provide prognostic information for chemotherapy: on the basis of certain clinical studies, it is now believed that women with 1-3 histologically positive axillary nodes may benefit from chemotherapy.

It is often the case, however, that no one treatment choice is optimal for all objectives. For example, WE is the least damaging cosmetically, but the chance of cure may not be as good as that of TM. TM with axillary dissection provides prognostic information for chemotherapy, but TM alone incurs less trauma.

2.7.3. Controversy

Historically, there has been bitter debate between proponents of different treatments. The radical mastectomy school felt that a surgeon must remove as much cancerous tissue as possible in order to prevent further spread of disease, and that "undue" consideration of cosmesis was an irresponsible action for a physician trying to save a woman's life. Another school of thought argued that in the absence of a demonstrated advantage to survival, consideration of cosmesis and surgical trauma was reasonable.

Clinical studies of varying quality fueled the fires of each side for some time. Finally the weight of evidence appeared to indicate that there was no survival difference between radical mastectomy and total mastectomy. But medical knowledge does not hold still, and the question today is whether total mastectomy might be replaced with wide excision. Here again, clinical studies are the critical basis which the clinician uses to decide which therapy is appropriate.

Chapter 3

Overview of the Research and the Roundsman System

This chapter presents an overview of the Roundsman project and the Roundsman computer program which is its central focus. Section 3.1 discusses an early stage of the Roundsman project: informal protocol analysis with an expert oncologist. Section 3.2 describes the development of a set of "scripts" which served as targets during program development and also helped to identify the set of publications which were incorporated into the Roundsman library (as described in section 3.3). Section 3.4 breifly presents the hardware and software which were used in program development. Section 3.5 outlines the steps taken by Roundsman when analyzing a case and then describes each of those steps in detail by tracing the execution of the system during an actual consultation.

3.1. Informal Protocol Analysis

How does a physician reason from the clinical literature? To gain insight into this question, the Roundsman project began with a period of informal protocol analysis. Previous work in medical protocol analysis has investigated diagnostic reasoning [Kassirer 82, Elstein 78] and has been particularly oriented toward causal models [Kuipers 84]. A senior oncologist at Stanford University Medical Center was asked to "think aloud" as he formulated management plans for primary breast cancer. These sessions were tape recorded and later analyzed. By varying the clinical studies which the oncologist could draw upon, it was possible to examine how a particular study contributed to the reasoning process, and how a study's role changed as additional studies were added to the "library". We were particularly interested in how the oncologist's *clinical judgment* affected the interpretation of statistical results and of the study as a whole.

Our investigation into how the expert oncologist uses experimental results clinically suggests that the critical reader embeds the results of a clinical experiment in contextual details "attached" to that particular study. These details help to interpret the meaning of the study's statistical results. These contextual details include:

- What type of patients seek care at the hospital where the research was done? To use the study as a basis for treatment, a physician must assess the differences between the study population and his own patient, and decide whether those differences are likely to influence outcome.

- What is the track record of the author? Have his previously published results been reproducible by other teams?

- How qualified are the allied specialties which are involved in patient care but are not the subject of investigation, for example post-operative nursing care?

- What are the exact technical details for the treatments being compared? (Two studies may compare the same drugs but the dose and dosing schedules might differ.) Before the study can be used as a basis for therapy planning, physicians must consider whether the technical approach used in the study differed significantly from the approach they are planning to take.

- How good is the biostatistical analysis?

An awareness of contextual details such as these allows the physician to decide how relevant the study is to his particular patient and treatment plan. The importance of this issue will be seen in the examples of Chapter 8; it also motivated the design of the "distance metric" described in Chapter 4.

Contextual details overlay the study's *experimental design.* The design may have significant complexity itself, and frequently requires analysis in assessing the study's relevance. For example, longitudinal, prospective comparisons of deliberate intervention [Bailar 84b] compare one therapy group to another *control* group which is optimally studied in parallel. Nevertheless, one of the most important sources of medical information has been the "case series" study, in which controls are external to the study (and therefore not formally matched at all).

Another dimension of design complexity concerns *stratification.* Patients are often sorted into strata according to variables thought to influence significantly their response to therapy. Results are then presented by stratum. Physicians can weed out many irrelevant tables and charts from the report if they can determine which stratum applies best to their patient. Even here however, the critical reader exercises clinical judgment. For example, if the strata were constructed after treatment ("post-stratification"), one must assess the investigator's intent: Was the stratification motivated by genuine clinical concerns or was it the product of a "fishing expedition" for a stratum that was statistically significant?

A viable model of the oncologists's behavior during these sessions then, is that clinical knowledge is structured around studies but in addition, also involves significant amounts of "contextual" knowledge which is often subjective in nature. This organizational view influenced the subsequent design of the Roundsman system. For example, in certain ways Roundsman's internal structures resemble a bibliographic retrieval system more than they resemble a traditional expert system.

That is, knowledge resides in separately identifiable "articles" rather than being merged into a knowledge base of clinical rules. There are large differences between Roundsman and bibliographic retrieval systems, but they do have in common the organization of knowledge around separate publications.

This publication-centered model, in which around studies as distinct entities, also allows the natural representation of *inter-study knowledge.* For example, study A might have had an irregularity in the experimental design which left some doubt as to generalizability of the main conclusions. Study B, published some time later, might demonstrate that the irregularity makes no difference, thus strengthening the principal conclusions of study A, even though it might have been designed to investigate a different question.

This section has described how the oncologist was observed to "critique" a proposed therapy for a particular patient by making reference to experimental study results in a the light of certain contextual details. Although this model of reasoning from the clinical literature has been outlined only roughly in this section, it can be seen to be quite different from causal modeling. Section 3.2 describes how target "scripts" were developed with the help of the oncologist. These scripts were developed following the period of informal protocol analysis described above, but *before* the development of a knowledge representation for the Roundsman computer program.

3.2. The Development of Target Scripts

To help design a computer program based on the publication-centered model, a set of "scripts" were developed in collaboration with the expert oncologist. These scripts served as targets for program performance. To obtain such a script a scenario was specified:

- A patient.
- A treatment proposal.
- A year. (The publications span several decades, but only those published prior to the indicated year were appropriate for discussion in the scenario.)
- A specification of relevant articles.

Six different scenarios were specified by varying the type of patient, the therapy decision, and the year in which the consultation takes place. The scripts were critiques of the relevance of the published studies to six clinical decisions.

For example, the scenario for script 4 is as follows:

- Patient: Tumor size of 1.5 centimeters, clinical node status N1b (palpable axillary nodes thought to contain tumor).

- Therapy proposal: Wide excision with axillary dissection, plus adjuvant radiotherapy.
- Year: 1977.
- Study cited in support: Peters67.

The script shown below begins with an introductory paragraph, proceeds to discuss each of these studies in some detail, and ends with a final paragraph summarizing the principal issues. (N.B. *This* script was produced by the investigator and domain expert, *not* by the Roundsman system.)

SCRIPT 4

The most relevant study for your decision is Hayward77. Peters77 is a later publication on the same population as Peters67, methodologically stronger than Peters67 because it adds matched control patients. Peters77, Guttman63 and Mustakallio72 are relevant to your decision, but less so than Hayward77.

Hayward77 reports the ten year results of a randomized trial at Guy's Hospital in England, comparing wide excision plus radiation to radical mastectomy plus radiation. The results showed a higher overall survival among Stage II patients in the radical mastectomy group. Although the difference was not significant at the .05 level, the authors did conclude that there was a suggestion that wide excision was not safe in stage II patients (like yours). A problem we are having with interpreting those results is that their radiation dose is suboptimal by today's standards for radiation therapy, and so your results might be better.

Peters77 is retrospective, case-control study comparing wide excision plus radiation to radical mastectomy plus radiation. We are having trouble applying the results to your patient for two reasons. First, your patient is clinical N1b and the study population is N0. Second, methodological flaws (the number of patients followed is not reported, and claims that aggressive surgery increased metastases causes us to suspect possible selection bias) make these results less useful than they might be.

Mustakallio72 uses external controls. In addition to this methodological weakness, the study population is clinical node status N0, unlike your patient who is N1b.

Guttman63 reports on a small number of patients with either excision or incision plus radiation, comparing them to external controls. Patients are stage II and III. It is significantly less relevant

```
(methodological weaknesses and different protocol than you propose)
than Hayward77.

There is reason for concern that for stage II patients like yours,
wide excision plus radiation is inferior to radical mastectomy plus
radiation. The radiation dose was suboptimal in Hayward77, but it is
nevertheless the best study to date. The other studies are less
relevant because their populations are different or their methodology
is weaker.
```

As mentioned earlier, these scripts were developed in light of the publication-centered view of the physician's knowledge, but *before* the development of a specific knowledge representation for either the studies or the contextual details. These scripts were judged to be strenuous performance goals for a novel type of computer-based advice, exhibiting a type of reasoning which had not previously been modeled in medical computer science. The Roundsman system's eventual output resembles the scripts fairly closely, although stylistic differences did evolve.

The six scripts also helped to identify publications which should be included in Roundsman's "library", as discussed in the next section.

3.3. Selection of Publications to Include in Roundsman

The publications which were eventually included in the Roundsman library were not screened according to whether they were the most methodologically "valid" in some absolute sense. (Indeed, in a system like Roundsman which is expected to know about, and comment on, any flaws, this is not necessary.) The studies were chosen because they had played a clinical role in the decades-old debate about the correct management of primary breast cancer. The collaborating oncologist has been clinically involved in this field for several decades. That made it possible to identify studies which, at key points over time, played an important clinical role in the debate.

For example, M.D. Anderson Hospital in Houston has an extremely large base of oncology patients. This significant "experience" with breast cancer patients gives Tapley's report from that institution [Tapley 82] a clinical importance despite many serious statistical weaknesses. A similar example is the experience of Dr. Haagensen from Columbia-Presbyterian Hospital, New York, who had as much personal experience with breast cancer surgery as any physician in the United States. When he published *case-series* reports of several hundred patients treated by radical mastectomy [Haagensen 63, Haagensen 69], these publications were clinically influential. (As the collaborating oncologist puts it, "those publications present the views of the most experienced expert in the field, buttressed with historical data.")

When more rigorous experiments were subsequently carried out [Fisher 80], they eclipsed the reports by Haagensen. But clinicians must regard the evidence as it presents itself.

Furthermore, some studies are considered methodologically valid at the time they are published, but *clinical* considerations that come into play later diminish the importance of the study. For example, the Guy's Hospital trial [Atkins 72] was a large, randomized trial of wide excision plus radiation versus radical mastectomy. It is difficult to fault the trial for statistical methodology: they did a superb job (especially for that time period). The results cast serious doubt on the safety of treating with wide excision and adjuvant radiation. However, in the course of this trial clinical thinking about the optimal dose of adjuvant radiation began changing. The Guy's protocol used a dose of approximately 2500 rads but during those years investigators began reporting that doses of 5000 rads were optimal. This reintroduced uncertainty: perhaps wide excision *could* be used safely with the increased radiation dose.

Roundsman's library includes 24 studies from 1948 to 1985. Full references for the publications can be found in the bibliography. A terse outline of the information represented by Roundsman for each study can be found in Appendix I.

3.4. Hardware and Software Support

The Roundsman system was developed on a Hewlett-Packard workstation (HP-9836) that is configured with 5 megabytes of RAM, a second independent color monitor screen and a 132-megabyte hard disk. This machine supports Portable Standard Lisp (PSL). Roundsman is written in GLISP [Novak 83] which provides the capability to translate to any one of several target LISP dialects (e.g., PSL). GLISP is an object-oriented language which uses partial data typing in order to pre-compile messages. This pre-compilation results in a faster run-time execution than that of many object-oriented languages.

3.5. An Overview of the Roundsman System

An outline of the steps taken by Roundsman when analyzing a case is provided below. Each step is described in detail later in this section.

1. Establish the "decision context". The decision context includes information about the patient and the therapy which the physician is proposing for that patient.

2. Focus on the class of questions most likely to interest the physician.

This entails deciding what types of therapeutic intervention should be compared. For example, in one time period it might be more appropriate for the machine to first discuss the surgical procedure, whereas in another time period it would be more appropriate to first discuss the use of (or omission of) adjuvant radiation with the proposed surgery. The need to establish an appropriate focus results because the clinical "consensus" changes over time, as discussed in more detail below.

3. Determine, for each study in the library, whether it can provide experimental results concerning that class of questions.
   If so, then

   a. Find the group (stratum) of patients within the study which most closely approximates the physician's patient.

   b. Identify any experimental results of that stratum which was treated with the interventions of interest (see step 2).

   c. Assess the "distances" between the physician's decision context and the particulars of the clinical study (see Chpt. 4).

   d. Return: the study results as applied to the chosen stratum, together with the distance assessments, to higher-level control functions in Roundsman. All this information is packaged in an object called a "datum-from-study".

4. Use the datum-from-study to compare alternative interventions on the basis of a model of choice and explanation (see Chpt. 5).

5. Pass the conclusions of the system to a prose generation module which assembles a prose critique for the user (see Chpt. 7).

An Example Prose Critique Generated by Roundsman

This section traces the execution of the Roundsman system during an actual consultation. In order to give the reader a clear understanding of the kind of critique the system is seeking to produce, Roundsman's output is provided below. The example is a verbatim transcript of Roundsman's critique of Veronesi81 *as it applies to*

- a 45 year-old pre-menopausal woman with a breast tumor 1.5 cm in diameter, clinically palpable axillary nodes suspected to contain malignant growth, and no known metastases (tumor growth in distant sites of the body), *for whom*

- wide excision surgery with adjuvant radiation has been suggested.

"Veronesi81 was a randomized, controlled trial carried out at the Cancer Institute in Milan. Patients were randomized to quadrantectomy combined with adjuvant radiotherapy combined with CMF for histology+ patients (N=352) or another protocol which was radical mastectomy combined with CMF for histology+ patients (N=349). Under the first protocol the overall survival at five years turned out to be 0.9 and recurrence-free survival at five years was 0.84. Under the second protocol the overall survival at five years was 0.9 and recurrence-free survival at five years was equal to 0.83.

"Are these results relevant to your patient? We suspect it makes little difference that the intervention was somewhat nonstandard (quadrantectomy removes more skin, fascia and muscle than wide excision). More troublesome is that first, the study protocol included a modality beyond your proposed treatment (chemotherapy was given if axillary nodes were histo+). Second, the study population was probably in a better prognostic stratum than your patient (they were clinically stage I).

"Reviewing the study itself, it helps that controls were randomly assigned (and stratified by menopausal status before randomization).

"Strictly on the basis of five-year results in recurrence-free survival, those two interventions look equivalent (the other results generally agree). The 'relevance' problems detailed above however, lead us to think that the results are indecisive for your purposes. Adhering to the standard of care (total mastectomy) would probably be most appropriate."

The remainder of this section traces how the critique was developed, following the five steps outlined above.

Establishing the Decision Context

To begin a session with Roundsman, the physician describes his patient and a treatment proposal through a process of menu selection. The description outlines clinical findings of interest to the management of primary breast cancer and is stored in Roundsman as an object of type *patient-description*, an example of which is shown in Table 3-1.

```
a PATIENT-DESCRIPTION with
     T-status = 'T1A
     N-status = 'N1B
     path-N-status = 'UNKNOWN
     M-status = 'M0
     age = 45
     menopause-status = 'PRE
```

Table 3-1: The *patient-description* object for the example session. The slots generic to this object type are shown in lowercase, to the left of the equals sign. The values for this patient are shown in uppercase, to the right of the equals sign.

The patient in this example has a breast tumor 1.5 cm in diameter, which falls into the breast tumor status T1a. She has clinically palpable homolateral (same side of the body as the breast mass) axillary nodes suspected to contain malignant growth which classifies her clinical node status as N1b. (Node status can also be determined by pathological exam but in this patient the path status is UNKNOWN.) The absence of known metastases (tumor growth in distant sites of the body) is metastasis status M0. All of this is stored internally as the *patient-description* object shown in Table 3-1.

```
an INTERVENTION with
 txtments = ( WE-WITH-AXILLARY-DISSECTION
              ADJUVANT-RADIATION-TX )
```

Table 3-2: The *intervention* object for this example session with Roundsman. The "txtments" slot has a value which is a list of objects of type *treatment*. The objects "we-with-axillary-dissection" and "adjuvant-radiation-tx" are subtypes of treatment, as shown in Table 3-3. The intervention object is more useful than a list of treatment objects because the Roundsman system can send high-level queries to the intervention object (e.g., whether it is a multi-modality intervention, how it is differs from another intervention) and let the intervenion object concern itself with computing the answer to these queries.

The physician proposes surgical wide excision plus axillary dissection combined with (post-operative) adjuvant radiotherapy. This is represented internally as the *intervention* object shown in Table 3-2. An intervention consists of a list of *treatment* objects. The Roundsman system has a hierarchy of treatments as shown in Table 3-3.

The *patient-description* and *intervention* objects are, in turn, components of the

- Treatment
    - Surgical-Procedure
        - Radical-Mastectomy
        - Total-Mastectomy
        - TM-With-Axillary-Dissection
        - Wide-Excision
        - WE-With-Axillary-Dissection
    - Radiation-Procedure
        - Adjuvant-Radiation-Tx
    - Chemotherapy
        - Adjuvant-Chemo
        - Adjuvant-Chemo-If-Histo-Pos

Table 3-3: The hierarchy of *treatment* objects known to Roundsman. Using this hierarchy, Roundsman can determine that the intervention shown in Table 3-2 includes a surgical procedure, a radiation procedure, and no chemotherapy.

larger *decision-context* object shown in Table 3-4. Roundsman uses this decision-context to dynamically assesses the relevance of a study to the patient and to the proposed intervention.

Focussing on a Class of Questions

Once the decision-context has been established, the system must decide what information is desired. To a certain degree this turns out to be a matter of user-modeling. That is, there is an enormous range of information contained in the clinical studies which is conceivably relevant. We have incorporated certain clinical heuristics which help to focus the system first on which issues are likely to be foremost in the minds of the user. This depends in large part on the clinical "consensus climate".

For example, in the contemporary (1986) climate of breast cancer management some clinicians might advocate surgical wide excision for this patient, but it is a controversial issue and total mastectomy is a more accepted surgical approach. Consequently, although Roundsman might discuss whether the user should have

```
a DECISION-CONTEXT with
   year = 1985
   subject-of-intervention =
      (a PATIENT-DESCRIPTION with
         T-status = 'T1A
         N-status = 'N1B
         path-N-status = 'UNKNOWN
         M-status = 'M0
         age = 45
         menopause-status = 'PRE)
   intervention-proposed =
      (an INTERVENTION with
         txtments = ( WE-WITH-AXILLARY-DISSECTION
                      ADJUVANT-RADIATION-TX ))
```

Table 3-4: The *decision-context* object for the example session with Roundsman.

This object is composed of a *patient-description*, an *intervention*, and the year of the consultation. The year is varied to investigate how the system's advice would "grow" over time. In a real system the year would of course be globally known to the program.

included radiotherapy (in addition to the suggested surgical wide excision), the collaborating oncologist feels that the discussion should first address the surgical choice itself and only secondarily address the question of adjuvant radiotherapy.

If the surgical choice is not clearly the "consensus" choice for that patient in that year, Roundsman first critiques the *surgical* choice. On the other hand, if the surgery proposed by the physician *is* the current treatment of choice for that patient, then Roundsman does not (as a first step) critique the user's surgical choice, but instead focusses on the physician's selection of (or omission of) adjuvant radiotherapy.

In the case being followed here, the surgery proposed (see Table 3-2 page 45) does not involve mastectomy, and Roundsman looks for information that would help decide between that approach and two classes of mastectomy: total mastectomy and radical mastectomy. The next two sections describe (a) how the system determines that Veronesi81 is pertinent to the case and (b) how it assesses the relevance of Veronesi81 to the physician's problem.

Searching a Study for Relevant Results

For this case, Roundsman has focussed on the question of non-mastectomy versus mastectomy. The system directs each study to determine whether it has experimental results concerning that question. At the implementation level this is accomplished by a series of message-passing operations. In order to make this process clear, the knowledge representation for studies is now discussed briefly. Following that, we resume a sequential discussion of the steps in Roundsman's execution (on page 49).

The Roundsman system is organized around frame-based data structures, some of which have been described above. A prominent data structure in Roundsman is the *study*. Veronesi81 is one of the studies represented in Roundsman's library.

The heart of each study consists of *comparisons* (sets of the data structure "comparison") and *strata* (sets of the data structure "stratum"), each of which is discussed below. In addition, each study contains certain descriptive information, such as the name of the institution where the research was carried out.

Each *comparison* contains knowledge about an experiment comparing one therapeutic intervention against another. For example, a schematic representation of one comparison from the Veronesi81 study is shown in Table 3-5.

```
 Intervention-A                          Intervention-B
 --------------                          --------------
Radical-Mastectomy                 We-With-Axillary-Dissection
Adjuvant-Chemo-If-Histo-Pos        Adjuvant-Radiation-Tx
                                   Adjuvant-Chemo-If-Histo-Pos
349  patients                      352  patients
RFS-5  = 0.83                      RFS-5  = 0.84
        standard error of the difference: 0.0396
        patient stratum concerned: 1
```

Table 3-5: An example *comparison* object from the Veronesi81 study. This is a schematic representation of the data structure.

The comparison in Table 3-5 encodes details about the *interventions* being compared, the *stratum* involved, and an *outcome* which was measured. It records the results of *recurrence-free survival* at five years (RFS-5). Another comparison might pertain to *overall survival* at five years. Each of these components (intervention, stratum, comparison) is, in turn, an object. For example, Roundsman has an *outcome* hierarchy in which "5 year survival" is one "measure of overall survival" (see Table 3-6).

Publications of clinical studies do not report data at the level of individual patients. A *stratum* is not a collection of patient records as in a data base, but is a summary description of a group of patients.

A stratum is much like a patient-description (see Table 3-1 page 45) except that

- Outcome
  - Measure-of-Overall-Survival
    - OAS-3
    - OAS-5
    - OAS-10
  - Measure-of-Recurrence-Free-Survival
    - RFS-3
    - RFS-5
    - RFS-10
  - Measure-of-Local-Regional-Recurrence-Free-Survival
    - LRRFS-5
    - LRRFS-10
    - IPSI-RFS-5
  - Measure-of-Distant-Recurrence-Free-Survival
    - DRFS-5
    - DRFS-10

Table 3-6: Hierarchy of *outcome* objects known to Roundsman.

```
     STRATUM

clinical stages:            (I)
tumor sizes:                (T1A T1B)
clinical node staging:      (NO)
pathologic node staging:    (UNKNOWN)
metastatic staging:         (MO)
menopausal status:          (PRE POST)
age-range:                  (20 . 70)
```

Table 3-7: Example *stratum* from Veronesi81.

since a stratum describes a *range* of patient types, the parameters of stratum may hold multiple values simultaneously. For example, a stratum from Veronesi81 is shown in Table 3-7. (Schematic descriptions of the system's knowledge for each study can be found in the Appendix I.) This stratum (Table 3-7) includes patients with either of two tumor statuses (T1a and T1b), a single clinical node status (N0), unknown axillary node pathology, no distant metastases (M0), both pre- and post-menopausal patients (PRE POST), and a wide age span (20 to 70).

To resume a sequential discussion of the steps in Roundsman's execution, the system directs each study to determine whether it has experimental results concerning the question at hand. This is implemented by message-passing operations. For example, comparison objects (see Table 3-5) can be asked (via message-passing) whether they involve comparing mastectomy to non-mastectomy.[1] Comparison objects in turn accomplish this by additional message-passing: they send messages to their constituent *intervention* objects, asking each whether they belong to a particular intervention class. The answers returned by the intervention objects allows the comparison object to answer the original question: whether it involves comparing mastectomy to non-mastectomy.

Those comparisons which are confirmed as pertaining to questions of interest are flagged, and the system then has statistical results of *potential* use to the physician. In this example, Veronesi81 is asked (via message passing) whether it can provide results of comparing a non-mastectomy approach to a mastectomy approach. As shown in Table 3-5, Veronesi81 does indeed have results relevant to that question.

The next step is to determine the stratum within Veronesi81 which most closely approximates the patient. Veronesi81 has only one stratum (see Appendix I) so the choice of stratum is trivial. However, when a study contains more than one stratum, Roundsman selects one of those on the basis of axillary node *pathology*. (Pathologic staging is more accurate than clinical staging, i.e., physical exam. Consequently, strata defined by pathology are preferred to strata defined by clinical staging.)

For example, if there were two strata, one with positive axillary node histology and one with negative histology, the system would conclude that the histologically positive stratum was most appropriate for the patient of Table 3-1 (page 45) since patients whose physical examination leads the physician to suspect tumor in the axillary nodes are more likely to have positive histology than negative histology. On the other hand, if strata were not defined histologically (i.e., pathologic node staging = UNKNOWN) then the system might attempt to find the most appropriate stratum based upon *clinical node staging* criteria.

As mentioned earlier, Veronesi81 has only one stratum, so that is clearly the "closest" stratum to the patient. There are two comparisons in Veronesi81 (see Appendix I for details), both of which pertain to the question of non-mastectomy versus mastectomy. Thus, these two comparisons are flagged for further consideration.

---

[1]The message is domain-independent; the arguments are domain-specific. For example, the system might send a comparison object the message "?do-you-contrast" with two arguments: <intervention-class-1> and <intervention-class-2>.

In this section we have described the outlines of the knowledge representation for studies, and traced how Roundsman identified Veronesi81 as pertinent to the case under consideration. The next section discusses how Roundsman assesses the relevance of Veronesi81 to the patient and treatment proposal.

Assessing Distance

If one could create a meaningful critique on statistical grounds alone, almost all of the knowledge about a study could be captured by the type of patients, the sample size, the interventions, and the outcome. As discussed in Chapter 4 however, these studies need more than an assessment of their *statistical validity* to be used productively in clinical reasoning. *They need clinical interpretation.* Roundsman would provide little of value if it offered merely a statistical skeleton as it's critique. Consequently, each comparison also possesses "distance metric knowledge" which is used to evaluate the clinical relevance of the statistical results to a particular patient and treatment, as described below.

Each *comparison* object which Roundsman uses in generating the critique has its own associated *distance metric* which is dynamically tailored to the patient and plan. This distance metric consists of a set of components which indicate how well the comparison applies to the patient and the proposed plan. This issue is discussed fully in Chapter 4. Here, a brief explanation of the process will suffice.

Distance metric components are one of three types: 1) population mismatches, 2) intervention mismatches and 3) methodological weaknesses. In the example session we are tracing, an example distance metric component (for an intervention mismatch) is shown in Table 3-8. In our example, the decision-context carries no suggestion of chemotherapy (see Table 3-4 page 47). In contrast, in the Veronesi81 study, chemotherapy was administered to patients who had positive axillary nodes by histological exam. This discrepancy is enough to trigger a distance-estimator to add the component shown in Table 3-8 to the distance between that study and the clinical decision begin analyzed. (One effect of this action can be seen in the second paragraph - third sentence - of the example critique shown on page 44.) Distance metric *components* therefore, are manipulated by *distance-estimators.*

Each *distance-estimator* contains clinical heuristics and judgments collected from our oncologist domain expert. A distance-estimator contributes to (and thus augments) the distance metric associated with a comparison, if the distance-estimator is triggered by an appropriate decision-context and study. The activation of a distance estimator results in the inclusion of a new component in the comparison's distance metric.

```
ADDITION-OF-BENEFICIAL-MODALITY  with

   dp-change = 'AWAY-FROM-ZERO-SMALL
   specifics = "chemotherapy was given if
                   axillary nodes were histo+"
```

Table 3-8: Example metric component: an *intervention-mismatch* object. Full explanation of the meaning and use of the slots "dp-change and "specifics" is deferred until Chapter 4.

In this manner, Roundsman's distance-estimators build up the distance metric of each pertinent comparison object. Each distance metric then contains a collection of the three component types: intervention mismatches, population mismatches and methodological weaknesses. After all such components are analyzed Roundsman uses them to assemble the example prose critique (page 44).

In what ways does Roundsman use the distance metric components when assembling a critique? The distance metric is used to identify the *character* of the issues involved in fitting a study to a clinical decision. For example, is the experimental design flawed or is this an otherwise good experiment which is difficult to apply to the physician's particular clinical situation? In the example critique, methodological issues are discussed separately from problems in applying the results to the physician's patient.

Distance information also allows Roundsman to identify the *magnitude* and *direction* of the component's effect. For example, the value of the "dp-change" slot shown in Table 3-8 contains a correction factor indicating the effect that this distance component has on the bare statistical results. One use of this information can be seen in the example critique: Roundsman groups serious problems separately from issues which are negligible. A full discussion of the distance metric is found in Chapter 4.

Comparing Alternatives

We have now traced through the first three of the five steps in Roundsman's operation. Step four, comparing alternative interventions, is accomplished via a *model of choice and explanation* which is the subject of Chapter 5, and is discussed briefly here.

Roundsman uses this model to draw conclusions about how alternative interventions compare to one another. These conclusions then serve as the basis for a prose discussion. For the example we are tracing, this prose discussion is the fourth paragraph of the example critique. It is important to point out that Roundsman's particular model of choice and explanation is really conceptually totally independent from its distance metric model. An entirely different approach to comparing alternatives might make equally good use of the distance metric.

Prose Generation

As mentioned earlier, Roundsman first draws its conclusions and then passes them to a text generation module which assembles the prose critique. The text generation module is called TEXTNET (an adaptation of PROSENET [Miller 84]), based on the "augmented transition network" (ATN) approach to natural language analysis [Woods 70, Miller 74].

TEXTNET is more flexible and expressive than "canned text" but less ambitious than computer science research projects in generating natural language [Weiner 80, McKeown 85]. Chapter 7 describes TEXTNET in terms generic to object-oriented programming. Chapter 7 therefore provides both (1) a description of Roundsman's text generation approach and (2) the information necessary for a system-builder to construct and use TEXTNET in any object-oriented programming language.

TEXTNET can be viewed as a collection of individual ATN's. Each ATN is responsible for describing to the user (in prose form) a particular subset of the system's conclusions. For example, certain ATN's discuss Roundsman's conclusions about how the alternatives compare to each other (the fourth paragraph of the example critique on page 44); other ATN's handle the discussion of methodological weaknesses, etc.

Chapter 4
Modeling Distance from Study to Decision

This chapter describes how Roundsman assesses the relevance of a clinical study to a physician's particular decision (step 3 in Fig. 1-1). Section 4.1 outlines Roundsman's representation of a study's statistical results: what interventions were compared, what outcomes were observed, etc. Section 4.2 presents a taxonomy of distances which allows Roundsman to *characterize* the distance(s) between study and clinical context. Section 4.3 describes the *calibration* of distance on a common scale. Section 4.4 describes the use of *distance-estimators* to identify when a particular distance metric component is applicable to the case being considered. Section 4.5 discusses related research, and section 4.6 summarizes the chapter's main points.

4.1. Representing a Study's Basic Statistical Results

Clinical studies report *outcomes* for particular processes under observation. Roundsman's studies report outcomes which are observed subsequent to *deliberate intervention* in the course of breast disease. (See "parallel studies of deliberate intervention" in Table 2-1, page 30.) These outcomes are merely the starting point for a useful evaluation of the clinical study. Roundsman must represent this information in a manner that allows the system dynamically to couple the statistical results with a critical assessment of their relevance to a clinical decision. This section describes how Roundsman represents these statistical results.

First, however, it is worth asking why statistical results should be separated from the clinical assessment of these results. Indeed, in an earlier stage of development, Roundsman's design did not make this separation explicit. *Relations*, in the predicate calculus sense, were the organizing element for the knowledge base. For example, the relation (BETTER total-mastectomy radical-mastectomy) stood for a study's principal implication. The support for this relation was encoded in a *justification* property which might include statistical results, knowledge about for which patients the relation was valid, reasons that the relation did not hold for other patient types, the degree of belief in the relation, etc.

The relation just described proved inadequate. First of all the relation does not clearly separate the oncologist's subjective knowledge from the recorded experimental observations. For example, the proportion of women observed alive after ten years in Hayward77 will not change, although the *subjective interpretation* of those results may well change. Expert systems which reason from heuristic knowledge or causal models do not have such a clear demarcation between "objective" facts and subjective judgment. (Many cause-effect relations and physiological models are treated as "fact" for a period of time, only to be invalidated and revised as new experimental evidence revises a theory of causality.) Reasoning from experimental evidence, on the other hand, clarifies the distinction between observed results and the subjective interpretation of those results. Consequently, Roundsman needs a representation which can accommodate these two levels of knowledge. The current implementation accomplishes this via a data structure called a *comparison*, and its associated *distance metric*.

A second reason that the relation scheme (described above) is inadequate is that it is meaningless to state that one treatment is better than another without specifying to which outcome and patient type the statement refers. For example, a treatment might be better for pre-menopausal patients but worse for post-menopausal patients. Likewise, a treatment might be better with respect to survival (one type of outcome) but worse with respect to the cosmetic damage incurred (another type of outcome).

As is outlined in Chapter 3, a *comparison* object is used to record the *statistical results* for each 4-tuple: (intervention-A, intervention-B, stratum, outcome-type). For example, one comparison instance might record *five-year* survival for intervention-A and intervention-B applied to a certain stratum. Another instance of the comparison object would be used for *ten-year* results. If there are two strata, then twice as many comparisons are needed to record the results. If there are three intervention arms, then comparisons are needed for A versus B, B versus C, and A versus C. The total number of comparison instances needed to encode the statistical results is equal to (# intervention-pairs) X (# strata) X (# outcome-types measured).

Two example *comparisons* are shown in Table 4-1. They encode statistical results observed on *stratum* 1 (the upper comparison) and *stratum* 3 (the lower comparison). The upper comparison records *recurrence-free* survival at five years while the lower one records *overall* survival at five years. They also compare somewhat different interventions: wide excision is used alone in the upper comparison while in the bottom comparison wide excision is combined with adjuvant radiotherapy.

As mentioned above and shown in Table 4-1, each comparison specifies *interventions* and *outcomes*. Because these interventions and outcomes are objects in Roundsman, the system can make inferences about a particular intervention and a particular outcome. An intervention consists of a set of *treatments*. Treatments belong to a treatment hierarchy. Similarly, *outcome* objects belong to an outcome hierarchy. Each *comparison* is linked to these hierarchies through its *interventions* and *outcomes*.

For example, the comparisons shown in Table 4-1 are linked to Roundsman's knowledge about treatments and outcomes as depicted in Fig. 4-1. Roundsman's

```
Tm-With-Axillary-Dissection         We-With-Axillary-Dissection
362  patients                       390  patients
RFS-5 = 0.72                        RFS-5 = 0.68
      standard error of the difference: 0.0495
      patient stratum concerned: 1


We-With-Axillary-Dissection         We-With-Axillary-Dissection
                                    Adjuvant-Radiation-Tx
358  patients                       373  patients
OAS-5 = 0.9                         OAS-5 = 0.91
      standard error of the difference: 0.0333
      patient stratum concerned: 3
```

Table 4-1: Example *comparisons* from Fisher85a.

Each *comparison* records the statistical results for a 4-tuple: (intervention-A, intervention-B, stratum, outcome-type). The upper *comparison* represents the five-year recurrence-free survival results for wide excision (with axillary dissection) versus total mastectomy (with axillary dissection). The standard error of the difference between proportions was calculated using life-table analysis and was provided in the publication. These results were observed for *stratum* 1 (each stratum in a study has an integer identifier). The lower comparison represents experimental results for somewhat different interventions and outcome types. The relationship of these two *comparisons* to other system knowledge is shown in Fig. 4-1.

outcome hierarchy allows the system to infer that comparison #1 concerns *recurrence-free* survival whereas comparison #2 concerns *overall* survival. Roundsman makes use of *overall* survival results in a different way than it makes use of *recurrence-free* survival results.

The treatment hierarchy allows Roundsman to determine which comparisons examine *adding* radiotherapy to a particular surgical approach (e.g., the lower comparison in Table 4-1), and which comparisons contrast *different* surgical approaches (e.g., the upper comparison in Table 4-1).

Comparison objects then, record the basic statistical results of an experiment. These statistical results are subjected to further assessment via *distance metric knowledge.* The statistical results can therefore by dynamically augmented with assessments made using this distance metric knowledge; they become coupled at run-time. The building blocks of that subjective assessment, *distance metric components,* are discussed in sections 4.2 and 4.3. The process by which these components are coupled with the comparison object (which contains the statistical results) is discussed in section 4.4.

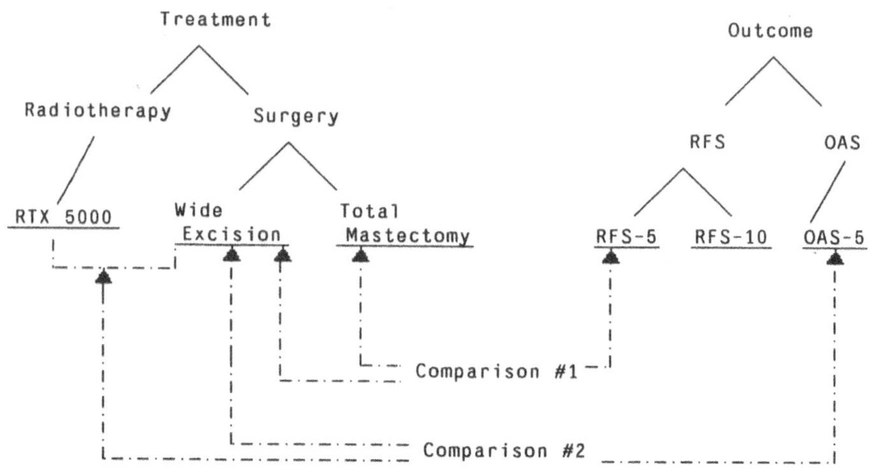

Figure 4-1: Comparisons are linked to treatments and outcomes. This diagram shows that comparison 1 holds five-year recurrence-free survival (RFS) results comparing wide excision *versus* total mastectomy. Comparison 2 holds five-year overall survival (OAS) results comparing wide excision combined with radiotherapy *versus* wide excision alone.

4.2. A Taxonomy of Distance

It is one thing to assign numbers to the distance from a study to a management decision. It is another to generate a critique which articulates the details of the distance assessment(s) in terms meaningful to the physician. In a medical advice system such as Roundsman, the results of the system are most likely to be used as a source of insight rather than as a final decision. Conveying the *semantics* of the judgments being made is central to the system design. The representation scheme for distance assessments must therefore be rich enough to characterize important types of mismatches.

For example, in breast cancer management, the patient's T (tumor) size might be larger than the study population's T size, implying that the study population may be in a better prognostic stratum. The system's critique must include details such as these so that the physician can understand the assessment and judge for himself how that factor should be interpreted.

Characterizing the semantics of a mismatch also helps in updating the knowledge base as new information appears. For example, in the 1970's total mastectomy was usually accompanied by radiotherapy: expert opinion held that radiotherapy was beneficial. When strong experimental evidence emerges which revises clinical opinion on that matter (e.g., [Fisher 80] demonstrated that radiotherapy has no benefit with respect to survival), it is important that Roundsman's now-obsolete distance assessment can be recognized and updated. Domain-specific details of the mismatch must be provided to the user so that obsolete interpretations can be recognized and updated, thereby helping to maintain the *integrity* of the knowledge base.

In matching a clinical study to a treatment choice, there are three general types of mismatch:

1. Differences between study protocol and the physician's treatment plan; this will be referred to as *intervention mismatch.*
2. Differences between the study population and the patient; this will be referred to as *population mismatch.*
3. Differences between the methodology used in the study and optimal methodology; this will be referred to as *methodological weakness.*

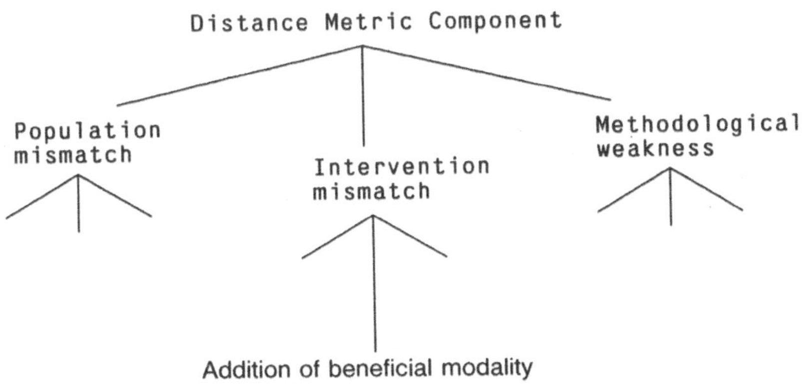

Figure 4-2: Partial hierarchy of distance metric components.
Distance metric components are one of three general classes: 1) population mismatch, 2) intervention mismatch or 3) methodological weakness. Each of these classes has subclasses. The figure shows one subclass of intervention mismatch. In the current implementation there are approximately 40 leaf nodes in this object hierarchy.

Methodological weakness is somewhat different in that it is internal to the study, while the other two types of mismatch refer also to the particular patient and clinical decision. However, in constructing the metric we deemed it desirable to have a uniform representation for components in the metric. Thus while this internal/external distinction is implicitly understood, it is not a criterion for creating separate representations.

These three general distance types have subtypes, and this hierarchy constitutes a *taxonomy* of distance metric components, as shown in Fig. 4-2. The branches underneath each of the three general types connote a bushy lower portion of the hierarchy. As an example, one member of the lower portion is shown explicitly: an "addition-of-beneficial-modality" distance metric component. This taxonomy, although developed for Roundsman, is not restricted to the domain of breast cancer: it is independent of that medical domain. The taxonomy provides a representation scheme for clinical studies, and may well provide a starting point for subsequent research aimed at modeling the process of reasoning from experimental evidence in other types of clinical literature.

Examples

To make Roundsman's distance taxonomy more concrete, we now enumerate certain of these distances, and provide examples from the domain of breast cancer management.

1. Better prognostic stratum

   - Class: population mismatch
   - Example 1: A recent article [Fisher 85a] is the best data on wide excision. The protocol in that paper specified that the margins of the excision had to be verified free of tumor by a pathologist before the patient was allowed into the wide excision group. (If the margins were not clear then the patient received a total mastectomy.) If Roundsman's user (a physician) does not have verification that the patient's excision margins were clear, then the study population is in a better prognostic stratum than the patient.
   - Example 2: If a patient has a large T (tumor) size, it is difficult to draw inferences from a study with a population of small T size.

2. Addition of beneficial modality

   - Class: intervention mismatch
   - Example 1: A proposed treatment plan of wide excision (alone) would be different from the protocol of the Guy's Hospital Trial

[Atkins 72, Hayward 77] which called for wide excision in combination with radiotherapy.

- Example 2: Fisher studied wide excision [Fisher 85a], but all patients with histologically positive axillary nodes also received chemotherapy. In critiquing a treatment plan to use wide excision, it would be important to point out that if axillary dissection reveals histologically positive axillary nodes, then only by adding chemotherapy would the treatment plan match the study protocol.

3. Lack of exclusion criteria

- Class: methodological weakness
- Example: After clinical studies have begun, it is not uncommon to find that certain patients refuse to accept the assigned therapy, or that some patients are ill with diseases unrelated to the study. The researchers may decide to exclude these patients from the analysis. The details of any such exclusions are crucial to a critique of the study. If these details are lacking, such a critique is greatly weakened.

4. Parallel non-randomized controls

- Class: methodological weakness
- Example: The patients studied Peters67 were not allocated to treatment groups randomly, but according to the wishes of the patient and her physician. This is a suboptimal experimental technique (as compared to randomization). For critiquing purposes, Roundsman's representation scheme must be able to express this judgment and *also* subtler distinctions. For example, one decade after the publication of Peters67, Vera Peters published Peters77. In this later study the controls were again non-randomized but treatment groups were *matched* by patient age, T (tumor) size and the year of treatment. Roundsman's critique must convey the oncologist's judgment that in comparison to Peters67, this matching strengthens the methodology even though it remains a non-randomized design.

5. Suboptimal therapy

- Class: intervention mismatch
- Example: In the context of wide excision, adjuvant radiotherapy dosages are currently in the range of 5000 rads. The 2500 rads used for the Guy's Hospital trials is (today) considered suboptimal.

6. External controls

    - Class: methodological weakness
    - Example: Levene77 reports on a case series of 64 women receiving biopsy combined with adjuvant radiotherapy. That is, there is only one treatment group; comparison to other treatment(s) is left to the reader.

7. Non-standard intervention

    - Class: intervention mismatch
    - Example 1: In the context of wide excision, the surgical protocol in Veronesi81 was "quadrantectomy" (removing a quadrant of the breast). This is a somewhat more extensive surgical procedure than wide excision (removing the tumor) but the oncologist feels that the survival difference would be insignificant. This judgment is a subjective clinical assessment.

8. Addition of useless modality

    - Class: intervention mismatch
    - Example: In the 1970's radiotherapy was routinely added to total mastectomies because it was believed to improve survival and to decrease the rate of local recurrence. Fisher80 and Fisher85b have shown that for certain patient groups it does neither of those things. Consequently, in 1985 a critique might mention that although the proposed treatment plan does not include the radiotherapy given in the study, this is unlikely to make any difference.

9. Non-specific protocol

    - Class: intervention mismatch
    - Example 1: The methods section of Hellman80 indicates that "some" patients had tumor removed by incision (taking a portion of the tumor), and some by excision (removing all tumor). Given this imprecision in the protocol it is difficult for a practicing physician to match the surgical approach.
    - Example 2: In G. Crile's studies, the "radical mastectomy" group only occasionally had chest wall musculature removed but more often the operation was closer to what is known as a total mastectomy. Few of the "radical mastectomy" group needed skin grafts, which is a typical part of Halstedian radical mastectomy.

10. Broad prognostic stratum

- Class: population mismatch
- Example: The patient is stage II, but the study was done on a stratum of *pooled* stage I, stage II and stage III.

11. Worse prognostic stratum

- Class: population mismatch

12. Immature results

- Class: methodological weakness
- Example: The average duration of followup in Fisher85a is 39 months. Many clinicians consider those results too premature to convincingly demonstrate survival results. This judgment is subjective and there is disagreement about how mature study results must be before applying them clinically. (Fisher's recent papers contain counterarguments against conservative MD's who won't believe results unless they are 10 years old. Fisher maintains that less mature results can be trusted.)

13. Selection bias

- Class: methodological weakness
- Example: During the 1950's and 1960's radical mastectomy was the standard of care. Total mastectomy was considered risky and experimental; it was undoubtedly quite difficult (politically) to justify an experiment comparing the two surgical procedures. Handley63 reports on a case series of 58 women treated with total mastectomy and radiotherapy. Handley writes, "selection for the operation [total mastectomy] was quite haphazard, and became more frequent as our confidence in the operation grew." Despite the understandable reasons for this approach to patient selection, it is the opinion of the expert oncologist that this selection bias makes the results of Handley63 somewhat less generalizable.

14. Poor follow up

- Class: methodological weakness
- Example: Patients enrolled in a clinical study may decide to move to another part of the country, or may simply lose contact with the hospital. The validity of the study depends on a vigorous effort to find out what happens to *all* of the patients enrolled. Or, if

certain patients are lost to "follow up" despite the investigators efforts, the study publication should address the question of whether the loss of those patients is likely to bias the results one way or the other.

15. Unreliable track record

- Class: methodological weakness
- Example: Studies from certain hospitals and investigators have not withstood the test of time. That is, results have not reproducible by others, and long-term results have been not been as good as would be expected by the earlier publications.

16. Temporal drift

- Class: methodological weakness
- Example: Mustakallio72 is one physician's report of twenty-five years experience treating breast cancer. The data are important, but the changes which have occurred during those twenty-five years (i.e., the nature of the disease and the technology of treatment) make it difficult to interpret this study for a clinical decision today. (The issue of interpreting oncology literature published some years earlier is discussed from a biostatistical perspective in [Feinstein 85].)

These "distances" constitute a vocabulary which applies across different studies, and is independent of the breast cancer domain. Indeed, it is a deliberate design decision to keep the taxonomy general enough that Roundsman's model might apply to various medical management domains. No "leaf" member of the taxonomy is refined further if that would create members of the taxonomy which are specific to breast cancer. All domain-specific information is restricted to three "properties" of taxonomy members: *specifics*, *dp-change* and *se-change*. The implementation of these three properties is discussed more fully below.

The distance taxonomy provides a way for Roundsman to accurately *characterize* the individual issues that make up the overall assessment of relevance. It also allows Roundsman to organize its discussion before printing the prose critique so that issues which are alike semantically can be discussed together. For example, in order to generate the prose output shown on page 44 of Chapter 3, the contributing metric components were first divided (dynamically) into two groups: (a) methodological weaknesses and (b) population mismatches or intervention mismatches. These two groups are then discussed in separate paragraphs.

The taxonomy is *implemented* in objects called *distance metric components*, two examples of which are shown in Table 4-2. Each distance metric *component* is an object in Roundsman. For each situation in which a particular type of distance is applicable, another *instance* of that object is created. The distance taxonomy allows Roundsman to determine what type of component it is handling (e.g., knowing that a component is a subtype of all classes above it in the taxonomy). Once Roundsman has decided how the critique will be organized, and where a particular distance issue will be discussed, the system can use two properties of distance metric components to produce text: the *general-declarative* property and the *specifics* property.

```
a LONG-ACCRUAL-PERIOD with
  specifics = "patient entry lasted from 1939 to 1972."
  se-change = INCREASE-SMALL
  dp-change = NONE


a BETTER-PROGNOSTIC-STRATUM with
  specifics = "they were clinically node negative"
  dp-change = AWAY-FROM-ZERO-MODERATE
  se-change = NONE
```

Table 4-2: Two "distance metric components".
The upper component is a *long accrual period* object, which is a type of methodological weakness (see Fig 4-2). The lower object is a type of population mismatch (see Fig 4-2). Slot names are to the left of the equals signs and slot values are to the right of the equals signs. "Specifics" is discussed in section 4.2. Both "se-change" and "dp-change" are discussed in section 4.3.

First, each distance component has a *general-declarative* text string which describes the general character of the component. For example, the general-declarative for the *long-accrual-period* object is "patients were accrued over a rather long period". That general-declarative is the same for all instances of the *long-accrual-period* object.

The *specifics* property of distance components is used to store a text comment that can be included in the critique. This text comment identifies the relevant "distance" issue more precisely than the distance metric component does by itself (see Table 4-2). Roundsman incorporates the *specifics* comment into the critique in whatever way the system-builder desires. (This is easily modified via TEXTNET, as described in Chapter 7.) Currently, the *specifics* remark is included as a parenthetical comment within a sentence that discusses the distance metric component. When adding distance metric knowledge to the system, providing "specifics" is optional. In generating a critique, if Roundsman makes use of a distance metric component which has no *specifics*, then the parenthetical remark is omitted.

For example, the expert oncologist might feel that a particular study's accrual period was longer than it ought to be. This judgment can be represented in the system's library by inclusion of a *long-accrual-period* object. Since the expert oncologist who makes this assessment is aware of study-specific details, he might well choose to include a more precise comment *within* that component, as shown in Table 4-2, to enhance the explanatory value of the critique.

The distance metric component shown in the lower half of Table 4-2 will, under the right circumstances, become a member of the distance metric for a certain *comparison* object. (The process by which these components are coupled with the comparison object is discussed in section 4.4.) Consequently, it would contribute to the critique. The *character* of this distance issue can be determined by the Roundsman system since the *better-prognostic-stratum* component is a machine-interpretable object, located under *population mismatch* in the distance taxonomy. Nevertheless, there is more than one situation in which the study population is from a *better-prognostic-stratum* than the patient. The *specifics* property carries a detailed remark, which can help to make clearer the source of this judgment.

The Roundsman system is able to identify the character of the remark contained in the *specifics* property (via the taxonomy) but that is the full extent of the system's knowledge about the remark (i.e., Roundsman does not "understand" the remark at all). In designing a system such as Roundsman, one might ask whether it would be better to identify the issues which are now embedded in the specifics remark, and explicitly represent them in yet another level at the bottom of the taxonomy. That is, would it improve the system to *refine* the taxonomy further?

It's true that this would provide a finer "grain size" for characterizing distance. For example, the *better-prognostic-stratum* object shown in Table 4-2 could be refined further so that *population-was-clinically-node-negative* is an object, but then the components are specific to breast cancer. This refinement has not been done in Roundsman because we want a knowledge representation which is independent of the breast cancer domain.

4.3. Calibration of Distance

The distance metric includes a measure of the size and direction of the mismatch. This aspect of the distance metric measures the *bias* of the study from the perspective of the clinical decision being made: whether a physician's plan is likely to have a better or worse outcome than the study population did, and by how much.

The primary goal of the Roundsman system is to identify the relevant issues and present them in a natural way so that the physician might make an informed decision. The numerical precision of the advice might be a second-stage (future) refinement on the model. Ultimately, even numerical estimates of distance must make some accommodation on the "grain-size" of the estimate. For example, it is unrealistic to use five significant figures if the expert oncologist is hard-pressed to assign more than one significant figure. The important point is not whether the current *implementation* uses the right level of precision, but whether the *model's* underlying scale for calibration is *ad hoc* (which would limit its extension to applications based on probability) or *formal*, with a well-understood interpretation within the scientific community. Roundsman's study results and distance metric are based explicitly on a probabilistic scale. Thus it could be extended or modified directly if more precise calibration were feasible and desired in another domain.

The studies in the Roundsman library report the *proportion* of women who are observed to have certain *outcomes* (e.g., five-year survival). Reporting proportions is common to many types of clinical studies. The central question asked in many longitudinal studies of deliberate intervention is, "Under which intervention does a larger *proportion* of the experimental subjects experience the outcome of interest?" For example, under which intervention do more women survive five years? A statistic of major interest is the *difference between proportions*, referred to here as *DP*. The value of DP lies between -1 and +1. (Each proportion lies between 0 and 1.) If DP = 0 then the observed proportions are equivalent, i.e., for the outcome under examination, the evidence demonstrates no difference between the two interventions. If DP > 0 then the proportion under intervention-A is larger than the proportion under intervention-B.

For example, assume the investigators in a clinical study observe that 60% of women treated by radical mastectomy survive five years, and 45% of women treated by total mastectomy survive five years. For this hypothetical example DP = (.6 - .45) = 0.15. The sign of DP depends upon the order in which the two interventions are considered.

The observed DP (0.15) is a *point-estimate* for the true DP. The *uncertainty* inherent in that estimate depends upon factors such as sample size. For example, one would be less certain of a point-estimate derived from observing 10 subjects than a point-estimate based upon observing 500 subjects. The point-estimate and the uncertainty can be both represented as a *probability density function* (pdf) over the range of possible values for DP. The mean of the pdf equals the observed DP (the point-estimate of 0.15, denoted DP†, pronounced "DP hat"). The shape of the curve indicates the degree of uncertainty: if the curve is "heaped up" so that most of the area under the curve lies close to DP†, then there is little uncertainty. Greater uncertainty is depicted as a curve which is more "spread out".

Since DP is a proportion, the pdf for DP† is a binomial distribution which can be

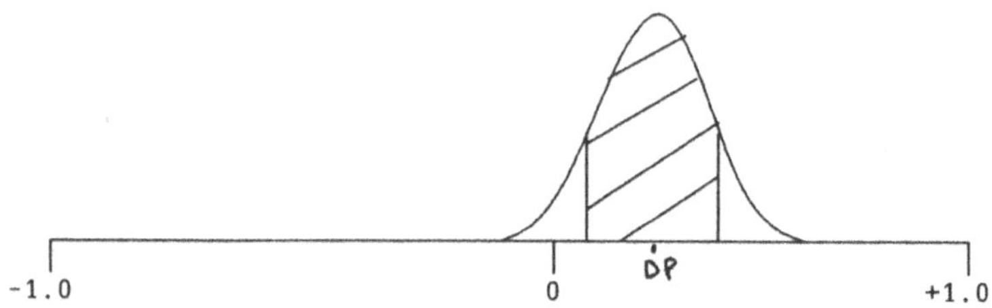

Figure 4-3: Probability density function (pdf) over DP.

This is a distribution over the difference between two proportions (DP). The mean is 0.15, and the spread of the pdf indicates the degree of uncertainty as to the exact value. The area between -1 SE and +1 SE is shaded.

reasonably approximated by the normal, or gaussian, distribution. The degree of "spread" for a gaussian distribution can be represented succinctly by the *standard error* (SE). Roughly two-thirds of the area under the pdf lies between $DP^{\dagger}$ - SE and $DP^{\dagger}$ + SE. Roughly 95% of the area under the pdf lies between $DP^{\dagger}$ - 2SE and $DP^{\dagger}$ + 2SE. An illustration of one such pdf is shown in Fig. 4-3.

The best initial estimate for $DP^{\dagger}$ is the observed difference in proportions reported in the study (DP). The initial estimate for SE is not quite as straightforward. If the authors of the study have used life-table analysis then the SE may be reported in the publication. If, on the other hand, the authors provide a SE for each observed proportion rather than the DP, then SE can be computed:

$$SE = \sqrt{(SE_{proportion\text{-}A})^2 + (SE_{proportion\text{-}B})^2}$$

If the authors do not provide a SE derived from life-table analysis then one might use Peto's estimate [Peto 77]:

$$SE = \sqrt{p_1(1-p_1)/r_1 + p_2(1-p_2)/r_2}$$

where p is the proportion of patients surviving in a treatment group and r is the total number of patients in a group.

Note that the estimate for SE incorporates only the sample size and the observed proportion. These statistics (observed proportion, sample size, SE) provide a *starting point* for interpretation of the clinical study. The effect of subsequent interpretation is represented as changes in the shape of the pdf: changes in the *location of* $DP^{\dagger}$ or the *size of SE.*

The expert oncologist may feel that a particular "distance" between study and clinical decision (i.e., patient and treatment plan) would change his best estimate for where the $DP^{\dagger}$ "should" really be located for the case at hand. In other words, he feels that the $DP^{\dagger}$ which is reported in the study must be shifted if it is to apply to a specific patient about whom a management decision must be made. One such shift in the location of $DP^{\dagger}$ is shown in Fig. 4-4.

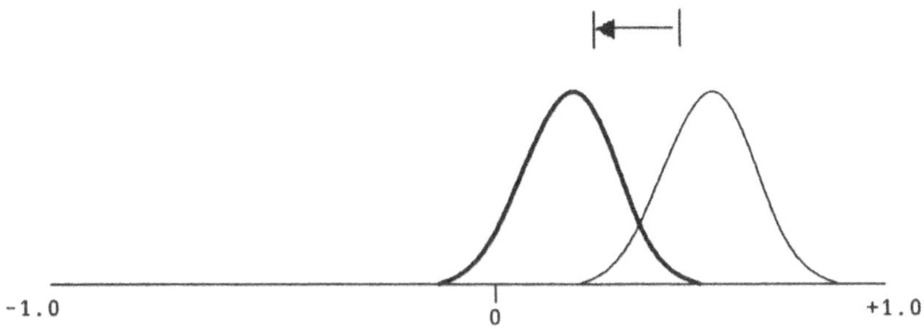

Figure 4-4: Illustration of a *DP-change.*

This figure shows a shift in the *location* of the best estimate for $DP^{\dagger}$. The shift indicates that, for this patient, the two treatments are expected to be more alike in outcome than they were in the study.

The *cause* of a shift is called an *absolute bias* or a *relative bias.* When the best estimate for $DP^{\dagger}$ in a particular patient is some *fraction* of the DP reported in the study, that is an example of a *relative* bias. The adjusted position of $DP^{\dagger}$ is the *product* of the prior DP and an adjustment factor. For example, there are situations in which the oncologist believes that the patient under consideration is less likely to die from breast disease within five years than the study population. (This could be due to a difference in clinical stage of disease.) Consequently, there is less opportunity for two treatments to demonstrate any differences they might have in curative capability. The oncologist's estimate for what $DP^{\dagger}$ should be is some fraction of the DP reported in the study. (If we were simply to *subtract* an adjustment factor, then if the study showed no difference between treatments the adjustment would incorrectly make one treatment look worse.)

An example of an *absolute bias* occurs when modernization of a treatment technique is believed to improve the outcome for one of two treatments examined in a study. The best estimate for DP† might therefore be the DP reported by the study plus a correction factor which accounts for the technological improvement. That is, the shift equals the algebraic *sum* of DP and an adjustment factor.

In the current implementation, Roundsman uses *rough estimates* of bias. For example, the following values of "DP-change" represent correction factors for *relative* bias:

- toward-zero-small
- away-from-zero-small
- toward-zero-moderate
- away-from-zero-moderate (see lower component in Fig. 4-2, page 65)

Again using rough estimates, Roundsman uses these values of "DP-change" to represent changes in location to correct for *absolute* bias:

- none (see top component in Fig. 4-2, page 65)
- negative-small
- positive-small
- negative-moderate
- positive-moderate
- negative-large
- positive-large

Distance(s) between study and clinical decision may also increase the *uncertainty* about what the true outcome will be. This is represented as a change in the size of the standard error (SE) of the probability density function (pdf). One such change in the SE is shown in Fig. 4-5. In the current implementation Roundsman uses these values for "se-change" to represent changes in the size of the SE :

- none (see bottom component in Fig. 4-2, page 65)
- negligible
- decrease-small
- increase-small (see top component in Fig. 4-2)
- decrease-moderate
- increase-moderate
- increase-extreme

<u>Correcting for Mismatch</u>

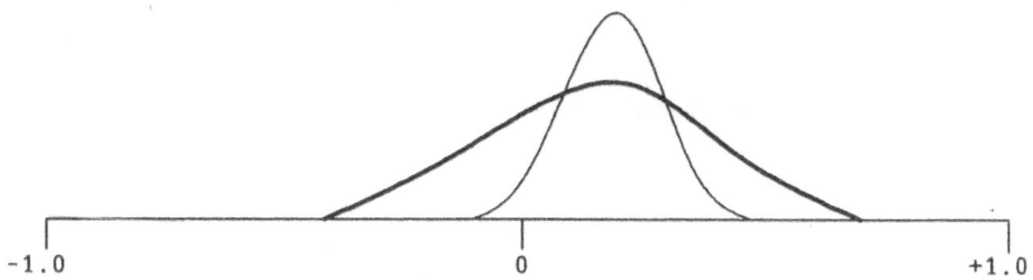

Figure 4-5: Illustration of an *SE-change.*
This shows a change in the size of the best estimate for SE. A particular clinical "distance" increases the uncertainty about what the outcome value will be. This is represented as a widening of the pdf. In this figure the location of the best estimate for DP† remains unchanged.

In critiquing a particular clinical decision, how might the system correct for a mismatch? The system might take two distinct types of approaches.

First, it might *transform* the study results, and offer advice as though the transformed study results were real data. That is, the system could shift the location of the pdf and change the SE of the pdf, and use the resulting curve for advice. It is important to note that this "debiasing" transformation is very inexact due to its subjective nature. So the results of "debiasing" should really allow only guarded comments of what the study implies with respect to the clinical decision at hand.[2]

A second approach would be to note the mismatch, and suggest a change in the clinical decision. For example, if unclear excision margins made study subjects ineligible for wide excision, the system might suggest pursuing the issue either to find out more about the patient's excision margins, or even to re-excise the tumor. This would *move the patient toward the study* population. As another example, if

---

[2]There is a technical difficulty that arises since the pdf lies between -1 and 1. If a pdf extends close to either of those borders, then increasing the SE (spreading the pdf curve) will overlap the border, which by definition it cannot do. This difficulty can be circumvented by mapping values within [-1, 1] to [$-\infty$, ∞] before manipulation of them. The function f=ln(1+x/1-x) accomplishes this. Increasing the SE along [$-\infty$, ∞] will not "run out of room". Several debiasing operations might be combined, cancelling each other if they are opposite in direction and size. Then $f^{-1}=(e^x - 1)/(e^x + 1)$ returns the curve to [-1, 1] for interpretation as a pdf over the DP.

radiotherapy was always part of the study's protocol, the system might point out that if radiotherapy were incorporated into the treatment plan it would be less difficult to confidently use the study results. This second approach to correcting mismatches highlights why it is essential for a system like Roundsman to characterize a mismatch as well as measure it.

The use of the correction factors (calibration values found in the "se-change" or "dp-change" slots") can be seen in the prose output shown in section 3.5 (page 44). In generating that critique, the relevant metric components were first divided (dynamically) according to whether they were (a) mismatches with the particular patient and treatment proposal or (b) methodological issues. This grouping is done via the taxonomy, not via the correction factors. Within the first group, components were further divided into three subgroups: good matches, mismatches that are negligible in overall impact, and mismatches that are significant. These three subgroups are sorted according to the seriousness of the mismatch as determined by the correction factors: "dp-change" and "se-change". Similarly, methodological issues were sorted into good methodology, methodological weaknesses of negligible impact, and serious weaknesses. Roundsman then assembled a prose critique in the context of those subdivisions.

4.4. Distance Estimators

The metric knowledge associated with a comparison consists of one or more *distance-estimators*. Each distance-estimator contains clinical judgments collected from our oncologist domain expert. Distance-estimators are capable of enlarging the distance metric associated with a *comparison*. For example, the distance-estimator shown in Table 4-3 would insert a "better prognostic stratum" distance component into the distance metric if, for the proposed treatment, a study population is in a better prognostic stratum than the physician's patient.

```
(a  POPULATION-DISTANCE-ESTIMATOR with

    outcome-eq-classes          = (OAS)
    intervention1-eq-classes    = (ANY)
    intervention2-eq-classes    = (ANY)
    study-pop-classes           = (T1-2 N0-1A)
    patient-classes             = (T1-2 N1B)
    bias-incurred   =
      (a BETTER-PROGNOSTIC-STRATUM with
       specifics = "they were clinically node negative"
       dp-change = AWAY-FROM-ZERO-MODERATE   ))
```

Table 4-3: A *population-distance-estimator* object.

The distance estimator in Table 4-3 lists "equivalence classes" which are defined on outcomes, interventions, population descriptions, and patient descriptions. The system has *population* distance estimators (to assess mismatches between a study population and a patient) and *intervention* distance estimators.

The population distance estimator shown above is activated if (a) the study stratum being examined by Roundsman is composed of subjects with tumor sizes T1 or T2, and clinical node status N0 or N1a, and (b) if the user's patient was tumor sizes T1 or T2 and clinical node status N1b. The estimated distance applies to outcomes within "OAS" (any "measure of overall survival"). The result of activating this distance-estimator is the insertion of a *better-prognostic-stratum* distance into that *comparisons* metric.

Some clinical "distance" issues are independent, while others are highly dependent. For example, in breast cancer management a patient with a large tumor size is more likely to show signs of involved nodes. That is, T (tumor) size and N (clinical node) status are highly dependent. This dependence is handled in Roundsman by explicitly grouping highly dependent parameters together in distance-estimators (as shown in Table 4-3). Additional examples of distance-estimators are provided in Appendix II.

Since the library of clinical studies is available *before* run-time, certain pre-processing of the distance estimators is done before run-time. Each distance-estimator searches the library for studies (and *comparisons* within the studies) which have the criteria which the distance-estimator requires before activation. It is not possible to know what the *decision-context* will be until run-time, but each distance-estimator builds up an index of relevant *studies* to which it could be applied beforehand.

4.5. Work Related to Roundsman's Distance Metric

This section contrasts Roundsman's use of "distance" to a variety of techniques which are peripherally related in potentially interesting ways.

Statistics: Regression Models

Logistic regression and proportional hazards regression [Cox 72] are biostatistical methodologies for analyzing the effect of covariates ("confounding variables") on an outcome of interest. Proportional hazards regression is often more appropriate when the outcome of interest is survival. Such a regression model will predict the change in survival expected from a given mismatch along some dimension such as size of tumor. One might ask, "Could a regression model drive the analysis which

Roundsman currently performs?"

Roundsman's distance metric model is, in fact, a sort of "heuristic regression model". (It is closer to statistical regression than it is to the AI work in analogical reasoning, which also seeks to measure a "distance" [Winston 75]. This may be because Roundsman and statistical approaches are interested in reasoning from experimental evidence, whereas the AI work in analogical reasoning has been concerned with distance between *concepts*.) But statistical regression is not quite the right tool for Roundsman for several reasons:

1. Publications often do not provide enough data to construct a regression model for the covariate causing the trouble. The publication may not provide a regression model which includes that covariate, and they seldom provide all the raw data for someone to construct a regression model from the publication. It is sometimes possible to get that raw data "released" by contacting the investigator personally, but more often it is not possible or is only attempted by individuals with specific *research* (rather than clinical) interests. The clinician must make do with what is available.

   There is currently discussion within the clinical trials community about including the raw data (on magnetic strips) as part of published papers. If this occurs, it will certainly improve the reader's access to data, but is unlikely to decrease controversy about its correct interpretation. Subjective clinical judgment will continue to be an element in the interpretation of biostatistical reports.

2. Statistical regression models are also unhelpful when there are no good data anywhere on the effect of a covariate. For example, for over a decade there was confusion about the correct interpretation of certain clinical studies comparing radical mastectomy and total mastectomy; the comparison of surgical alternatives was muddied by the fact that radiotherapy was added to one or both of the surgical procedures. There were no data available to construct a regression model to analyze the separate effect of adjuvant radiation (especially for total mastectomy). The judgments were subjective, based upon soft data.

   A second example of this absence of data is the important investigation which employed quadrantectomy as the "non-mastectomy" intervention [Veronesi 81]. (For an explanation of the differences between local excision and quadrantectomy, see Fig. 2-1, page 33.) There is no real way to know if quadrantectomy results should be used to make inferences about wide excision.

Another problem is that several of the distance assessments are supra-study, like "highly-respected-author". These are some of the situations in which Roundsman uses a physician's subjective clinical judgment.

3. Finally, statistical regression would not be helpful in *characterizing* the type of mismatch. That is not a criticism of regression: the technique is not intended to do that. But this capability is important for Roundsman in order to discuss the basis of the analysis in its critique.

Decision Theory: the DEALE Model

The DEALE model is an approach to estimating a patient's life expectancy [Beck 82]. The DEALE model is directed at estimating life expectancy for a given clinical situation but it is not particularly suited to comparing alternative interventions, (nor was that the purpose of the model). The DEALE model requires that mortality rates be available for the age, sex, and race of the patient and the disease process being considered. When the clinical decision involves controversial treatments, however, those rates are unknown. The DEALE model is pertinent to Roundsman because it might help correct for coexisting diseases.

A study designed to compare two treatments for a particular disease often disqualifies patients with coexisting diseases. For example, most studies of breast cancer patients exclude patients with a prior malignancy. Also, any patient with heart or lung disease is usually excluded since these disorders might put the patient at high risk during surgery.

Consequently, recommending therapy for a patient with one of these other problems can be difficult. If the coexisting disease has no obvious interaction with breast cancer or the treatments being considered, the DEALE model might be an excellent way to adjust for the coexisting disease. Roundsman does not implement such considerations, however, in its current version.

Artificial Intelligence in Legal Reasoning

Law is based in part on the principle of "stare decisis", the doctrine of precedent, which includes citing and arguing from precedents. For example, lawyers may establish analogies with those precedents favorable to their client's position, and differentiate their client's position from precedents that do not favor their client.

Some researchers maintain that the key to creative legal reasoning is quite unlike case-based reasoning, and their work emphasizes other aspects [Gardner 84]. However, it is relevant to mention AI research which explores case-based reasoning in law: the HYPO project.

The HYPO system [Rissland 85] contains a knowledge base of past legal cases. The goals of the system are (a) to identify legal precedents which can be cited to support arguments in favor of the client and (b) to point out arguments which might be made by the opposing lawyer, and weaknesses in those arguments. A legal case is represented by frames, and the slots are called "dimensions". By permuting the details of a precedent, creating hypothetical precedents, the HYPO system explores ways to strengthen or weaken the client's argument. Starting with the case at hand and varying the values of dimensions, the system tries to produce hypothetical legal cases ("hypos") and searches for matchings in the knowledge base.

From the critiquing perspective, HYPO and Roundsman share certain objectives. Also, in the same way that shifting the background of precedents with HYPOS gives law students more practice around one case, creating fictitious clinical studies might allow medical students to learn how to explore reasoning from the clinical literature.

There are, however, major differences between legal reasoning and clinical reasoning from experimental evidence. As a result the design of the Roundsman system is quite different from that of the HYPO system. In the scientific paradigm, one assumes that the investigation is in search of an unique underlying (biologic) truth. Interpreting clinical trials is evaluating *experimental evidence*, and statistical theory is central. As the following quotation from [Gardner 84] makes clear, solving legal problems is quite different:

> There is no hidden reality [in legal reasoning] to be discovered or, remaining undiscovered, to be 'covered for'; the question is how to characterize the reality that is known. Accordingly, probability theory is not just limited, but inapplicable.

Unlike legal precedents, clinical studies are not gold standards: they are imperfect *experimental evidence*. Roundsman must deal with the weaknesses of clinical studies as experiments.

Another difference is that in legal debate, false arguments may have value to one party. For example, among the rhetorical techniques which interest one legal reasoning researcher [Rissland 85] are "obfuscating", and "minimizing exposure" to facts which weaken the argument. HYPO project researchers are currently examining the applicability of the game-theory paradigm to legal argument: in order to plan a strategy, HYPO might "look ahead" at all the possible moves and counter-moves of the two legal teams. The emphasis is on placing the case in the right light, rather than on sharpening one's perception of an underlying "reality".

4.6. Summary

The model used by the Roundsman system includes two types of knowledge about clinical studies: (a) basic statistical information such as the treatments compared, the outcomes observed, and (b) subjective clinical judgments about the *distance* of the study from different decision contexts. The *comparison* object and its associated *distance metric* allow these two types of information to be separately encoded.

Components of the distance metric are members of a *taxonomy* which is independent of the breast cancer domain. The distance taxonomy allows Roundsman to characterize the issues of interpretation in order to generate a critique. Domain-specific information is embedded in one or more properties of a distance metric component. The taxonomy provides a representation scheme for subjective interpretation of clinical studies. It may well provide a starting point for subsequent research aimed at modeling the process of reasoning from experimental evidence in different types of clinical literature.

Chapter 5
Choice and Explanation

This chapter discusses Roundsman's approach to evaluating alternatives (step four of Fig. 1-1). Sections 5.1 through 5.9 present the conceptual basis of this step, a multiattribute model of choice and explanation. Section 5.10 describes the implementation of that model in Roundsman. The final section outlines key features of the model and summarizes its implementation in the Roundsman system.

It is important to understand the relationship of this model of choice and explanation to Roundsman's distance metric model described in Chapter 4. The distance metric model is *independent* of the approach taken to choice and explanation. This independence is advantageous: entirely different approaches to comparing alternatives might nevertheless use the same distance metric model.

5.1. Introduction

Within artificial intelligence (AI) research, programs developed to assist medical *diagnosis* have been characterized along a number of dimensions. For example, diagnostic programs have been analyzed as subtypes of classification problem solving [Clancey 84b]. Comparisons have been drawn about their handling of uncertainty [Szolovits 78], and whether their representation is adequate for explanations [Hasling 84]. Medical *management*, on the other hand, has not been as well characterized; few unifying concepts have been identified.

This chapter outlines a model of choice and explanation in medical management, identifying its advantages and limitations. The model is based on multiattribute decision making (MADM) [Hwang 81, Keeney 76] and consists of four distinct strategies for choice and explanation, plus combinations of these four. Each strategy is a restricted form of the general MADM approach, and each makes restrictive assumptions about the nature of the domain. The four strategies therefore cannot be seen as "general problem solvers". Rather they are techniques which allow a general solution (MADM) to be fitted to a domain. The advantage of tailoring a general technique to a particular domain in a restricted form is that it may better capture the character of the domain and allow choice and explanation to be more naturally modelled.

The use of the strategies for both choice and explanation are illustrated below with examples from the management of primary breast cancer, and are also described in the setting of several existing medical management AI systems. Using the model it is possible to identify common underlying features of those systems, since they each can be seen to have employed portions of the model in different ways. Thus the model lets us better understand and characterize the seemingly ad hoc decision making approaches used in these previous systems.

Whenever possible, multiattribute utility terminology is used to characterize these AI systems, all of which have been observed to perform at the level of experts to some degree. It is important to keep in mind however, that this chapter is superimposing a multiattribute model on systems which were not designed with specific utility characterizations in mind. Consequently, there is bound to be a certain degree of haziness in the assumptions of some of these systems. The intent of this chapter is:

- To make certain aspects of these previous systems clearer by using a multiattribute model to analyze them. This will hopefully make these important AI systems more accessible to a decision analytic audience and, at the same time, suggest ways in which AI researchers might design systems in which assumptions are represented more explicitly.

- To present a multiattribute model that can be used by the Roundsman system for choice and explanation in the current domain of application: the choice of a surgical and radiotherapeutic plan for the management of primary breast cancer.

5.2. Multiattribute Decision Making

The model borrows concepts from the field of multiattribute decision making (MADM). Management choices (for example, choice O and choice O') are characterized by n-tuples in which each entry (v_i) is the value of an attribute (i). Throughout this chapter we use 3 attributes for simplicity of exposition, although the analysis would of course generalize to n-tuples of any size n.

$$O : (v_1, v_2, v_3)$$
$$O' : (v_1', v_2', v_3')$$

For example, if O and O' are choices for the management of primary breast cancer then v_1 might be the value of the attribute "5-year survival rate", v_2 might be the value of the attribute "cosmetic damage", and v_3 might be the value of the attribute "trauma of the procedure".

In order to compare two choices and decide which is superior, one must somehow estimate the value of the two n-tuples, reflecting the overall desirability of each. *Value functions* of this sort are not new to AI. For example, most chess-playing programs use an evaluation function that maps the characteristics of a move into a scalar value. This scalar is then used to compare the desirability of moves. Decision theory makes use of a similar construct, the utility function U, which maps into the zero-one range:

$$U(v_1,\ v_2,\ v_3) \dashrightarrow [0,1].$$

In decision theory there is a formal distinction between utility functions and value functions. This is not important for the purposes of this chapter, however, and the more familiar term "utility function" will be used here in a general sense.

Utility functions can be quite complex, and their construction is non-trivial. As a result the more complex models are frequently difficult to explain. An elaborate decision model may obscure the salient features of the problem, trading off an ability to explain choice in intuitive terms in favor of achieving a more powerful, generalized characterization of the problem. A comprehensive treatment of utility models in multiattribute decision theory has been written by Keeney [Keeney 76]. Multiattribute decision theory is the subject of an excellent survey by Hwang [Hwang 81] and a special issue of *Management Science* [Spronk 84].

Analysis of previous AI research in medical management suggests that there are common structures underlying the seemingly ad hoc solutions used by these systems for choosing therapy. As this chapter describes, the concepts of multiattribute decision making can be used to interpret these AI programs. A further application domain, the management of primary breast cancer, is used to show how four strategies derived from MADM can all be illustrated in a single medical domain, as well as in these several previous systems.

5.3. The Importance of Modelling Both Choice and Explanation

In medical management it is common for there to be more than one correct way to manage the patient. Users of advice systems for medical management can be expected to demand a reasoned argument for the system's choice [Teach 81]. A model of medical management should therefore be able to deal with both choice *and* explanation. Because of this need to model explanation as well as choice, a system builder may find that a *general solution* to selecting optimal treatment (e.g., the axioms of utility theory, with no other assumptions, constitute one general approach that can be applied to *any* domain) may not be the best solution to use for a specific domain. Modeling a particular treatment decision frequently does not need the full power of the general approach. Furthermore a general model may not lend itself to terse and concise explanation.

This chapter shows how four comparison strategies, each of which is a restricted version of MADM, may allow a system builder to tailor the general MADM approach to a particular domain. The use of the more restricted strategy may allow more concise explanation, and (as we will show) may even capture more naturally the character of the choice itself.

5.4. Four Strategies for Choice and Explanation

In the model we include the four strategies itemized below, *and* combinations of them.

- Lexicographical ordering
- Satisficing
- Dominance
- Trade Off

These four capture the decision-making character of those systems we analyzed. There may be other strategies, but these four are a useful set to build upon when examining other domains whose decision-making character has not been rigorously analyzed. Each of these strategies will be described in terms of MADM. Each makes restrictive assumptions as to the nature of the domain. Thus, each is a restrictive version of a general approach (MADM). As described above, the advantage of using these restricted versions of the general approach is that choice and explanation may be more naturally captured.

Two of these strategies (lexicographical ordering and satisficing) require strong assumptions, as discussed below. Each strategy may be reasonable for different domains. Combinations of these strategies have been used in MYCIN, EXPERT/CASNET and the Digitalis Therapy Advisor. They are well suited for management of primary breast cancer as well. When the strategies are applicable, better explanations may be possible *because* the strategies entail stronger assumptions (i.e., more knowledge of the domain).

5.5. Lexicographical Ordering

5.5.1. Operational Definition

$$O : (v_1, v_2, v_3)$$
$$O' : (v_1', v_2', v_3')$$

All four strategies involve first establishing a "rank-ordering" of values v_i within each attribute i (e.g., v_1 is preferred to v_1'). Lexicographical ordering further imposes a strict ordering on the attributes themselves (e.g., attribute 1 is more important than attribute 2 etc.). Choices are then compared attribute-by-attribute. If one choice is superior based on the most important attribute, then the process halts. Tying choices are carried forward to be compared on the next attribute. As a result, this strategy assumes that even a small preference on the most important attribute outweighs all the less important attributes. This is clearly a very strong assumption. The term lexicographical ordering is used since this technique is analogous to a dictionary which is ordered lexicographically by the letters in each word.

5.5.2. Examples

Management of Breast Cancer

In developing a system to advise in the management of primary breast cancer, we have worked in collaboration with one of Stanford University's senior breast cancer specialists. He evaluates five attributes of a management choice (Table 5-1).

1. chance of cure
2. cosmetic damage
3. trauma of the procedure
4. chance of local recurrence (breast or chest wall)
5. prognostic information for chemotherapy

Table 5-1: Attributes used for choice of therapy in primary breast cancer.

Furthermore, the oncologist clearly uses lexicographical ordering in making management choices. When deciding between therapy options, he first looks at the chance of cure. If one alternative is best on this attribute, then he will choose that alternative. (The differences must be statistically significant; i.e., the evidence, however imperfect, must suggest that there is a meaningful difference.) If more than one alternative is "tied" for best on chance of cure, then he eliminates all other alternatives and carries those that tie forward, to be considered on attributes such as cosmetic cost and trauma of procedure. Those attributes are considered using approaches other than lexicographical ordering. Thus he essentially divides the attributes into "chance of cure" and "all other attributes", using lexicographical ordering to make a unique choice or to eliminate some alternatives before consideration of "all other".

Note that this use of lexicographical ordering tells us a great deal about the attributes in this domain. No combination of values on cosmetic cost and trauma of procedure can "make up for" a loss on chance of cure. In another domain this might not be the case. But it appears to be the case in this domain, and we can take advantage of this for choice and, as is shown later, for explanation.

The Precedence Scheme of EXPERT

EXPERT is a domain-independent tool for building expert systems; it was first applied to diagnosis and therapy selection in ophthalmology [Weiss 78]. An approach to therapy selection developed for EXPERT was called the *precedence scheme* [Kastner 83]. This approach evolved from Kastner's experience with limitations of a rule-based approach to treatment selection. He viewed the precedence scheme as possessing several advantages:

> "The simplicity and elegance of the treatment selection scheme has enabled our medical collaborators to specify their method of choosing treatments easily. This scheme has provided a concise formalism to encode therapy planning knowledge ... One of our medical collaborators now teaches his students ... using this formalism." [Kastner 83] (page 47)

> "Often a large number of production rules can be rewritten as just one precedence rule. Furthermore, the precedence rule is computationally more efficient in both storage and time than the corresponding set of production rules ... In addition the scheme is simple enough that the consequences of a change have typically been readily apparent." [Kastner 83] (page 48-49)

> "The precedence scheme provides several explanation capabilities. The system can produce the rationale behind the choice of treatment. In addition, the ranking of the alternative choices of treatment is explained and comparisons between any pair of alternative treatments can be produced." [Kastner 83] (page 48)

The precedence scheme is organized in the form of charts, where each column is labelled with a drug choice. These choices are sorted by an "a priori consideration", for example the efficacy of the drug against ocular herpes virus. Thus the most efficacious choice is at the far left, and the least efficacious at the far right (Fig. 5-1). Rows are labelled with other considerations, for example contraindications to treatment with that drug such as (1) a patient being allergic to the drug, or (2) pregnancy when the drug is known to be dangerous in pregnancy. Rows are also arranged in order of importance, with the most important row on top. For example, in Kastner's charts the "severe allergy" row is above the "mild allergy" row (as "contraindication1" is above "contraindication2" in Fig 5-1). Checks are inserted in the chart to indicate that the drug in that column is relatively contraindicated for the patient.

Processing of the chart is accomplished by repeatedly sorting and resorting the list of drug choices. The procedure sorts by rows, starting with the bottom row and moving up gradually to the top row. At each row a re-sorting occurs: if a column has a "check" under it, then that column is moved to the far right end of the drug list. When the process is complete, the preferred drug choice is in the left-most column.

	drug1	drug2	drug3
contraindication1			√
contraindication2	√		
contraindication3		√	

Figure 5-1: The precedence scheme developed for EXPERT.
In this somewhat simplified illustration of the precedence scheme developed for EXPERT, check-marks indicate that the drug in that column is relatively contraindicated for the patient.

Kastner argues that

> "Precedence rules provide a new way to express knowledge that heretofore was either specially coded in general purpose language or was represented by many unrelated production rules." [Kastner 83] (page 111)

Kastner's precedence scheme can be viewed as an implementation of lexicographical ordering. Let the rows each be attributes, and the initial column position be the value of another attribute. As mentioned above, in many examples rows represent contraindications and the initial column positions represent an ordering by drug efficacy. In Fig. 5-1 the initial position of drug1 is the leftmost column, indicating that it is considered the most efficacious. The strict ordering of attributes is as follows: contraindication1 before contraindication2, then contraindication3, and finally efficacy (which is defined by initial column ordering rather than by an additional row at the bottom of the chart). Kastner separates drug efficacy from the other attributes, calling this the "rationale behind ordering". Rationale-behind-ordering may be conceptually separate from contraindications in a medical sense, but with respect to an abstract evaluation function it can be modelled simply as another attribute.

Lexicographical ordering requires that attributes be strictly ordered and that preference among choices can be determined by comparing attributes in order, independently of other attributes. The precedence scheme obeys both requirements. The assumptions of lexicographical ordering are recognized by Kastner:

> The sort procedure requires a few assumptions of the disease model. The ordering of importance of the sort keys [attributes] must be strict. For instance, in this case resistance is a more important factor than allergy. No interdependencies between or combinations of the keys is considered. [Kastner 81] (page 909)

Because of these assumptions, new attributes (e.g., additional contraindications) can be added without modifying other attributes. Kastner extends the precedence scheme to merging therapies [Kastner 83] (i.e., combining treatments for a multiple disease diagnosis). It can be shown that this is also an example of a lexicographical evaluation function.

5.5.3. Assumptions

Lexicographical ordering assumes that no combination of later (less important) attribute values can "make up for" even a small loss on an earlier (more important) attribute. That is, if the attributes are ordered 1 before 2 before 3,

$$U(v_1, v_2, v_3) > U(v_1', v_2', v_3') \quad \textit{iff}$$

$$v_1 > v_1'$$

$$\text{or } v_1 = v_1' \text{ and } v_2 > v_2'$$

$$\text{or } v_1 = v_1', v_2 = v_2' \text{ and } v_3 > v_3'$$

5.5.4. Explanation

If lexicographical ordering is applicable, explanation of the system's choice can be intuitive and succinct. *Question:* "Why did you recommend total mastectomy and not wide excision with axillary dissection and radiotherapy ?" *Response:* "Because total mastectomy provides a better chance of cure." It is not necessary to refer to the relative value of cosmetic loss as compared to chance of cure, and how the overall utility scores evolved. Moreover, that kind of explanation would be incorrect: it does not reflect how the decision was made.

5.6. Satisficing

5.6.1. Operational Definition

$$O : (v_1, v_2, v_3)$$
$$O' : (v_1', v_2', v_3')$$

Satisficing again requires establishing a rank-ordering of values within each attribute. Next one designates a "satisfactory level" s_i for each attribute i. If $v_i < s_i$ choice O will be eliminated from contention. Thus satisficing involves establishing a *threshold* of acceptability for each attribute. Note that satisficing becomes meaningless if no choice meets the threshold value.

5.6.2. Examples

Management of Breast Cancer

Chemotherapy has been shown to be of benefit to women with 1-3 histologically positive axillary nodes. Because of this, the collaborating oncologist satisfices on attribute 5 of Table 5-1 ("prognostic information for chemotherapy"). He eliminates from consideration any therapy choice that does not include prognostic information for chemotherapy advice. (Such information is usually obtained by axillary dissection. If a diagnostic test is developed which provides the same prognostic information, however, then axillary node dissection might be dropped from the treatment of primary breast cancer.)

MYCIN's Revised Therapy Algorithm

Although MYCIN is often described as a diagnostic program, its principal motivation was to assist with selection of therapy [Buchanan 84]. MYCIN's diagnostic phase identifies several organisms, one or more of which may be causing the infection, and which must therefore be treated with antibiotics. At this point the diagnostic phase has been completed but the non-trivial problem of therapy selection remains:

> "The main problem of the therapy selector is to prescribe the best drug for each organism thought to be a likely cause of the infection, while minimizing the total number of drugs. These two constraints often conflict: the best prescription for, say, four items may require four different drugs, although for any patient usually no more than two drugs need to be given (or should be, for reasons of drug interaction, toxic side effects, cost, etc.)" [Clancey 84c] (page 134)

Clancey found the rule-based format a difficult representation for design of a therapy selection algorithm:

> "We found it increasingly difficult to keep records during the program execution for later use in the explanation system; indeed, the logic of the program was too confusing to explain easily. We decided to start over, aiming for a more structured algorithm that would provide sophisticated therapy, and by its very organization would provide simple explanations for a naive user." [Clancey 84c] (page 134)

The revised therapy algorithm developed by Clancey considers five goals (Table 5-2). These concerns which guide MYCIN's revised therapy algorithm are called "goals", "constraints", "local considerations", "global considerations" and "criteria" at various times [Clancey 84c]. They can also be seen as the attributes of a multiattribute decision problem, whose solution is a mixture of two strategies: trade-off and satisficing. Goals 1 and 2 are used to generate a list of candidate drug therapies, and will be discussed later when trade-off approaches are considered. Each candidate solution is then tested (using a generate-and-test paradigm) against goals 3, 4 and 5. The algorithm therefore *satisfices* on goals 3, 4 and 5 and the first candidate to achieve satisfactory levels (i.e., "true") on all three becomes the recommended therapy. (There are subtleties to MYCIN's assessment of contraindications, and how likely an organism must be to warrant therapy, but these capabilities can be ignored for purposes of the current discussion.) This example is a "degenerate" case of satisficing since only "true" and "false" values are used. Satisficing is a more general strategy that can also be used with a continuous-valued attribute.

1. Use the most effective drug for each organism.
2. Use the fewest total drugs
3. Treat all of the likely organisms
4. Avoid the selection of two drugs from the same drug class (when their effects are redundant)
5. Avoid drugs to which the patient is allergic or which will cause harm

Table 5-2: Goals of the MYCIN revised therapy algorithm.

5.6.3. Assumptions

For each attribute there is some minimum satisfactory value which an alternative *must* achieve in order for the choice to be acceptable, i.e., this is a class of utility functions such that $U(v_1, v_2, v_3) = 0$ *iff* $v_i < s_i$ for any i.

Note that satisficing does not take into account how "close" v_i is to the threshold s_i.

5.6.4. Explanation

When satisficing applies, it is possible to provide better explanation of choice by taking advantage of the stronger assumptions. *Question:* "Why didn't you recommend total mastectomy or total mastectomy plus radiotherapy?" *Response:* "Neither of those procedures would provide prognostic information for advising the patient about chemotherapy." It is not necessary to refer to the relative value of various attributes, and how the overall utility scores evolved. An explanation that included discussion of inter-attribute weighting or overall utility would miss the essential nature of the decision. Satisficing seems to be a domain-independent abstraction for the medical notion of "absolute contraindication".

5.7. Dominance

5.7.1. Operational Definition

$$O : (v_1, v_2, v_3)$$
$$O' : (v_1', v_2', v_3')$$

As with the previous strategies, dominance requires establishing a rank-ordering of values within each attribute.

O *dominates* O' *iff*

$$v_i \geq v_i' \text{ for all i,}$$
and
$$v_i > v_i' \text{ for at least one i.}$$

In other words, for a choice to be superior to another choice by dominance, it must be clearly superior on at least one attribute, and at least tied on all others.

Dominance and satisficing might be seen as "special cases" of lexicographical ordering. That is, if option-1 *dominates* option-2 then certainly option-1 would also be preferred under lexicographical ordering. The point is that satisficing and dominance each give us another view of the nature of the decision. These views are useful for explanation.

5.7.2. Examples

Management of Breast Cancer

Dominance is a most useful strategy for explanation of choice. The following example shows how dominance can be used to choose between radical mastectomy (RM) and total mastectomy with axillary dissection (TM+axilla). RM appears to provide equivalent chance of cure as TM+axilla, and the chance of local recurrence is also equal. Both of these choices provide the prognostic information necessary for chemotherapy advice. TM+axilla is a less traumatic surgical procedure, and the cosmetic results are better than RM. Thus, with respect to the five attributes just mentioned, TM+axilla *dominates* RM.

MYCIN's revised therapy algorithm

After MYCIN has offered therapy recommendations, the user may ask why a particular therapy was *not* recommended. MYCIN would respond by explaining why the recommended therapy was superior to that alternative. For example, one transcript (see Figure 6-9 of Buchanan and Shortliffe [Buchanan 84]) shows the user asking MYCIN why it did not recommend an alternative drug combination. MYCIN notes that the recommended therapy is, drug-for-drug, more efficacious (attribute 1 in Table 5-2) than the alternative and furthermore that the two therapies are equivalent with respect to the total number of drugs (attribute 2) and the contraindications (attributes 3, 4 and 5).

5.7.3. Assumptions

The only assumption of the dominance relation is that the utility function is well behaved, i.e., if $v_i \geq v_i'$ for each i, then $U(v_1, v_2, v_3) \geq U(v_1', v_2', v_3')$ for any v_i, v_i'. This is a reasonably safe assumption.

5.7.4. Explanation

Dominance is intuitively persuasive in explanation. *Question:* "Why did you recommend total mastectomy with axillary dissection rather than radical mastectomy?" *Response:* "Because total mastectomy with axillary dissection is better than radical mastectomy with respect to cosmetic costs and trauma of the procedure, and the two approaches are otherwise equivalent." This explanation does not require any inter-attribute comparison.

It is anticipated that in the domain of breast cancer management there will seldom be a single dominating alternative. As a result, a unique choice can seldom be made solely by dominance. There may, however, be a set of dominated alternatives and a set of *non-dominated* alternatives. Treatment choice can then be made from the non-dominated set. Even if a *recommended* choice cannot be selected by dominance, however, dominance may still be useful for explanation if a question is asked as to why a dominated choice was *not* recommended.

5.8. Trade-Off

5.8.1. Operational Definition

$$O : (v_1, v_2, v_3)$$
$$O' : (v_1', v_2', v_3')$$

Here again, one must first establish rank-ordering of values within each attribute. Then one incrementally converts O and O' such that they differ only in one "surviving" attribute. For example, one might convert various morbidities into dollars or into "quality adjusted life years" (QALYs).

If one performs a trade-off with full knowledge of the exact *values* of the attributes, then one might have enough information to figure out the relative "weights" of the attributes in terms of each other. That is, one might convert O' (shown above) by exchanging v_3' for v_3 plus an "offset" of k_a in the same units as v_1'. The converted $O' = ([1+k_a]v_1', v_2', v_3)$. A similar exchange of v_2' for v_2 plus an offset of k_b yields $O' = ([1+k_a+k_b]v_1', v_2, v_3)$. Now O and O' differ only in the first attribute. Since there exists a rank-ordering within this surviving attribute, choice is now straightforward. Note that this trade-off is assessed *locally* for pre-enumerated choices. If all possible choices can be pre-enumerated when building an advice system, then trade-offs might be done at design time.

If there are too many choices to enumerate them all (and perform trade-off) while building the system, then one needs a general algorithm to make the trade-offs dynamically. A utility function such as $U(v_1, v_2, v_3) = v_1 + a \cdot v_2 + b \cdot v_3$ (a restricted version of the additive form) can be viewed as encoding the trade-off between attributes. More complex general forms such as multiplicative utility functions are sometimes better approximations of the real world, but so difficult to assess that additive forms are used anyway. Another difficulty is utility dependence among attributes. For example if the decision-maker's utilities are examined closely it may become apparent that the decision maker's relative "weighting" of v_2 and v_3 could change as the value of v_1 changes. A complex utility function is needed to represent this behavior (see Keeney and Raiffa [Keeney 76] for a full treatment of this topic). It is eventually necessary to compromise between oversimplification and complexity of the model.

5.8.2. Examples

Management of Breast Cancer

If the oncologist cannot make a choice based upon chance of cure, and cannot select a unique choice by satisficing on prognostic information, then he is forced to consider the trade-offs between goals 2, 3 and 4 (Table 5-1). [The choice being made here is the surgical approach. The choice of whether to use adjuvant chemotherapy would involve trade-off much more prominently.]

MYCIN's Revised Therapy Algorithm

As described previously in the section on satisficing, MYCIN uses goal 1 from Table 5-2 ("use the most effective drug for each organism") and goal 2 ("use the fewest total drugs") to generate a list of candidate drug therapies. This phase of the algorithm involves *trading-off* between *effectiveness* and *total number* of drugs. In other words, the dependence between these two attributes is handled via trade-off. Choosing the most effective drug for each organism (attribute-1) takes priority as long as the number of drugs (attribute-2) is two or fewer. But then the goal of keeping the number of drugs small begins to "make up" for a drop in effectiveness. Thus it is seen as optimal to trade-off attribute-1 in order to improve on attribute-2. This trade-off solution is encoded implicitly in the algorithm which generates candidate solutions.

The details of this trade-off are as follows. For *each* suspected organism, drugs are placed into rank-1, rank-2 or rank-3, according to the drug's effectiveness against the organism. This process is repeated for all organisms that must be treated. The result is that there is a set of antimicrobial drugs in each of three "bins": rank-1, rank-2 and rank-3. Note that the same drug may appear in more than one bin, because it may be an excellent drug for one organism (going into rank-1) and less effective against another organism (going into rank-3). The algorithm then generates a list of candidate solutions (a list of sets of drugs) in order of decreasing desirability:

all solutions of the form ($DRUG_{rank-1}$)

...

all solutions of the form ($DRUG_{rank-1}$, $DRUG_{rank-1}$)

...

all solutions of the form ($DRUG_{rank-1}$, $DRUG_{rank-2}$)

...

all solutions of the form ($DRUG_{rank-1}$, $DRUG_{rank-3}$)

...

In this way the *trade-off* between effectiveness and total number of drugs is encoded implicitly. These candidate solutions are then tested by satisficing on goals 3, 4 and 5, as described previously.

The Digitalis Therapy Advisor: ANNA

The Digitalis Therapy Advisor [Silverman 75, Gorry 78] is a program designed to help physicians prescribe a dose of the drug digitalis for particular patients. This program uses body weight, age, target blood concentration and other parameters of a pharmacokinetic model to produce an initial dose estimate. Subsequent feedback about toxic and therapeutic states (qualitative information) then guides adjustments to these parameters of the pharmacokinetic model. For example, one parameter is the "body stores goal". The Digitalis Therapy Advisor's combination of mathematical modeling and AI techniques was novel, as was its emphasis on feedback about the patient's response to earlier therapeutic actions. For therapy choice, the system determines to which of nine "patient response classes" the patient belongs; the dimensions of this classification are level of toxicity and therapeutic response. Treatment actions (in the form of recipes) are associated with each of these nine classes.

Toxicity and therapeutic response can be viewed as attributes of a multiattribute decision. In this system, the trade-off between all possible values of toxicity and therapeutic response has been determined *a priori* in constructing the actions attached to each of the nine patient response classes. As soon as the values of those two attributes are known, the choice of therapy action is automatic; this reflects the fact that the designers have predetermined an adjustment to parameters of the pharmacokinetic model.

ATTENDING

ATTENDING is designed to critique an anesthetist's plan for premedication, induction, intubation and maintenance of anesthesia [Miller 83b, Miller 84]. The central data structure is a hierarchy of augmented transition networks (ATNs). The system searches this hierarchical planning network in order to identify alternatives to the user's proposed plan, comparing the risks of the user's proposed arc (action) to the risks of parallel arcs. ATTENDING considers only one attribute: risk. Benefits are handled as negative risks. Risk takes on one of four values: Low, Moderate, High and Extreme. The system dynamically identifies the path through the net which corresponds to the user's proposed plan, and then it examines alternative paths. These paths have a set of risk values that are assigned by considering the particular patient's clinical context for each of the therapeutic actions that make up the path, e.g., "medium", "low", "high", "medium", "medium". In comparing two paths then, the system must compare two *sets* of risk values.

Risk is the surviving attribute of a trade-off performed at the time of system design. The choices have been pre-enumerated, and trade-off assessments made so that choices differ from each other in only one attribute. For example, another design might represent "avoidance of hepatotoxicity" and "avoidance of bronchospasm" as explicit attributes. The values of these attributes would be the expert's estimate of how well a particular anesthetic avoids hepatotoxicity and avoids bronchospasm. (e.g., Halothane-induced hepatotoxicity is a clinical concern. With respect to bronchospasm, halothane is a bronchodilator and thus may help avoid bronchospasm.) However, in ATTENDING all attributes have been traded off so that only one attribute remains: Risk. The system is then able to compare choices along this single dimension. A single risk value may incorporate *several* individual morbidities, each with an (implicit) probability and utility. In other words, the values of *risk* represent $\sum$ P(morbidity$_i$) * U(morbidity$_i$). Folding severity and probability together makes it somewhat difficult to characterize the assumptions of ATTENDING from a decision theoretic perspective.

5.8.3. Assumptions

There are no strong assumptions necessary to use the trade-off strategy. In fact, it can be thought of as a general fallback technique. If the assumptions of the other strategies are not reasonable in a domain of application, one can use trade-off.

Summary of the Strategies

- Lexicographical Ordering: O is preferred to O' iff $v_i > v_i'$ where i is the first attribute in which O and O' differ, when attributes are examined in the pre-specified order. For example, if attributes are ordered 1 before 2 before 3,

$$U(v_1, v_2, v_3) > U(v_1', v_2', v_3') \quad \textit{iff}$$

$$\begin{aligned} & v_1 > v_1' \\ \text{or } & v_1 = v_1' \text{ and } v_2 > v_2' \\ \text{or } & v_1 = v_1', v_2 = v_2' \text{ and } v_3 > v_3' \end{aligned}$$

- Satisficing: There is a threshold value of attribute i below which any choice O is considered unacceptable. That is, given threshold level s_i for attribute i, $U(v_1, v_2, v_3) = 0$ *iff* $v_i < s_i$ for any i.

- Dominance: O *dominates* O' *iff* $v_i \geq v_i'$ for all i, and $v_i > v_i'$ for at least one i.

- Trade-Off: O is preferred to O' if you can find a mapping such that O and O' differ in only one attribute v_i, and $v_i > v_i'$.

Table 5-3: Summary of multiattribute interpretation of the strategies. This table outlines the strategies in terms of two choices O and O', where O $= (v_1, v_2, v_3)$ and O' $= (v_1', v_2', v_3')$.

5.8.4. Explanation

Explanation of trade-off may be more difficult than with the other strategies, but unavoidable if the character of the domain is such that the other strategies do not apply. The nature of the explanation will depend on the nature of the trade-off which has been made. If the trade-offs are not discussed in detail the system can only offer a superficial explanation, which merely mentions the attributes involved. *Question:* "Why did you recommend adjuvant radiotherapy in combination with the wide excision procedure?" *Response:* "Although radiotherapy does incur some additional trauma and transient cosmetic damage, our assessment is that these are outweighed by the benefit of reducing the chance of local recurrence in the breast."

5.9. Comparison Strategies Under Uncertainty

The previous discussion has ignored decision making's probabilistic element. This is a crucial point, because medical management decisions are often probabilistic. Our analysis of previous work shows that the four strategies might also be applied to medical management under uncertainty.

The probability distribution over a binary outcome might itself be viewed as an attribute value. For example, in breast cancer management there is a probability distribution for the outcome "five year survival". This is a binary outcome: patients either survive five years or they do not. The mean of this distribution can be viewed as the value of an attribute called "P(survive-5-years)".

The practice of discretizing a probability distribution can be seen in several of the systems mentioned above:

- In MYCIN the probability of killing organism_j with drug_k, which is a probability distribution if modeled in full detail, was represented as one of four values for $\text{"effectiveness"}_{j_k}$. Effectiveness is an attribute with possible values of "rank-1", "rank-2", "rank-3", or "none".

- In the CASNET/EXPERT system there is concern about allergic reactions. In CASNET this was modelled as three values: "mildly allergic", "moderately allergic" or "severely allergic". Since CASNET was not designed in terms of an explicit multiattribute model, it is not clear whether these three values discretize the probability of allergy, or whether they represent an amalgam of the *probability* of an allergic reaction and the *utility* of such a reaction: P(allergic reaction) * U(allergic reaction).

- The ATTENDING system uses one attribute, called *risk*, with values "low", "moderate", "high" and "extreme". As mentioned above, this single risk value may incorporate *several* individual morbidities, each with an (implicit) probability and utility.

In each of these examples some information is lost. For example, one such loss is the variance of the distribution on $P(\text{killing organism}_j \mid \text{drug}_k)$ in MYCIN. There are arguments for being more exact by including the variance:

- Risk aversion: In decision theory, one can characterize how averse a decision maker is to taking risks. For example, a decision maker might not agree to pay \$10 to buy a 50-50 gamble on \$100. He is considered "risk averse" because the expected value of such a purchase is profitable, but he did not want to take the risk of losing \$10. Risk aversion makes a large variance less desirable, even if the mean outcome is the same.

- Value of information: There exists some disagreement about the applicability of "second-order distributions" on probabilities used in decision theoretic models. Nevertheless, the use of a density function to represent the decision-maker's knowledge about a value between 0 and 1 is embraced by many Bayesians [Howard 70, Doubilet 85, Critchfield 86]. The crux of the issue is whether or not there is an opportunity to gather more information on the decision. If there is any opportunity to learn more, then it is quite important that the representation for, say P(5-year survival), be able to reflect variability. It is the feeling of many Bayesians that *in the real world* there is almost always an opportunity to learn more about the decision, and that probabilities are more usefully represented as density functions than point estimates.

Of course exact solutions are frequently not possible, and are not always necessary. In any case, in practical decision support systems it may be more important to identify the risks, to include them in approximate calculations, and to be capable of *explaining* their implications.

In addition, there are typically some attributes for which uncertainty is minimal. For example, consider the attributes in management of breast cancer (Table 5-1). Given a management choice, the second, third and fifth are known with virtual certainty while the first and fourth are highly uncertain. In situations like this, the comparison strategies mentioned earlier could be very useful. For example, *satisficing* on prognostic information is entirely possible, regardless of any uncertainty on the first and fourth attributes. Similarly, if *lexicographical ordering* models a domain, and the non-probabilistic attributes are ordered first, then a decision might be made on lexicographical ordering without requiring that the system process the probabilistic attributes at all.

5.10. Implementation in Roundsman

This section describes Roundsman's implementation of the multiattribute model described in the previous sections of this chapter. This analysis produces certain inferences which are then used by TEXTNET in creating the prose critique. The last paragraph of the example critique in Chapter 1 serves to illustrate how Roundsman uses the model of choice and explanation:

> "Strictly on the basis of five-year results in recurrence-free survival, those two interventions look equivalent (the other results generally agree). The 'relevance' problems detailed above however, lead us to think that the results are indecisive for your purposes. Adhering to the standard of care (total mastectomy) would probably be most appropriate."

That paragraph of prose critique is based in large part upon the conclusions drawn from choosing lexicographically, using the "cure" attribute. Cure is an important issue in breast cancer management, and assessment of the cure *attribute* by Roundsman is correspondingly a central component of its analysis. For this reason, much of this section concerns Roundsman's assessment of cure. Before discussing that attribute more fully, we first review Roundsman's basic approach to evaluating alternatives.

As described in sections 1-9 of this chapter, our oncologist compares alternative treatments in roughly the following way:

1. *Satisficing* on the prognostic information obtained by axillary node dissection. (The oncologist rejects any treatment option that does not include axillary node dissection.) This issue emerged in the early 1970's when it became known that axillary node information could help predict the efficacy of chemotherapy for women with breast cancer.

2. *Lexicographical ordering* on the basis of cure. If a treatment is superior on cure, that treatment is chosen[3]. As will be discussed below, assessing the value of the "cure" attribute is not necessarily clear-cut. Deferring this issue for the moment, it can be said that *if* the clinician feels that the evidence demonstrates *equivalent* curative potential between the alternatives, he will then consider trade-offs between issues other than cure (see step 3 below).

3. *Trade-off* between cosmetic costs, the trauma of the procedure, and the chance of local recurrence (see Table 5-1, page 83).

Lexicographical Ordering on "Cure"

In comparing alternative interventions, Roundsman looks at which alternative is most likely to cure the patient. This assessment involves a great deal of clinical judgment: there are many outcomes which are *indicators* of cure, but no single, unambiguous measure of cure. For example, our collaborating oncologist feels that

---

[3]When the character of the domain changes, the strategy of choice may change as well. For example, the choice of adjuvant chemotherapy, which is outside the scope of Roundsman, involves more consideration of the trade-offs between cure and the various side effects of the drugs.

recurrence-free survival data are a better indicator of cure than *overall survival.* (Overall survival includes women in whom cancer has re-surfaced but who are still alive.) The time course of breast cancer is long: five, ten or even fifteen years may elapse before the patient succumbs to the disease. Consequently, the proportion of patients alive at three or five years may not accurately reflect the curative value of an operation, whereas the proportion free from *any* recurrence of their disease may be a better indication of ultimate results. Thus the domain of oncology is markedly different from say, acute respiratory failure (e.g., respiratory distress syndrome) where the patient either recuperates or dies within a few days or weeks.

In addition to different *outcomes* (e.g., overall versus recurrence-free survival), the clinician assessing a study on breast cancer must also decide what *duration of follow-up* is adequate. As mentioned earlier, after five years of follow-up not all women who will *eventually* succumb have died. Some of the best investigators in breast cancer management argue that five year results are robust enough to compare the curative value of therapies [Fisher 85b]. Most clinicians are more conservative: they hesitate to rely on five-year results, and prefer to wait until ten year results are available. Indeed, certain breast cancer surgeons will rely only on results with a maturity of fifteen years.[4] This caution stems from the character of the domain: breast cancer is a disease with serious consequences.

The life-and-death character of breast cancer also influences choice in another way: clinicians exhibit a strong tendency to adhere to the current "consensus" treatment unless the evidence favoring another treatment is very solid. The conservatism about new treatments reflects the nature of the domain. This conservatism might not be true in choosing a drug to treat high blood pressure. In that domain, one might find physicians much more willing to alter their choice of treatment based upon tentative evidence that one drug is better than another.

Roundsman assesses cure via empirical evidence in the form of reported *outcomes,* such as the proportion of women surviving five years. Each of these outcomes might be seen as *subattributes* in a hierarchy of attributes. For example, in a hierarchy of attributes, five and ten-year survival would be subattributes of cure. A separate subattribute would be necessary to encode whether a treatment is currently the "consensus" choice in the clinical community. In order to incorporate all of these considerations into the assessment of cure, one might develop a model which

---

[4]The pros and cons of using outcomes such as five and ten-year survival for clinical decisions are discussed from a decision-theoretic viewpoint in [McNeil 78]. In this book, it is not my purpose either to question or to defend this aspect of clinical decision-making in oncology.

"weights" the subattributes. There are in fact many reasonable approaches to combining subattributes in order to obtain the value of the parent attribute. (Attribute hierarchies has been described in decision theory [Keeney 76] and in computer science research [Wellman 85].) In many ways this is a system design issue: the multiattribute representation can always be made more elaborate if this additional development effort would help to meet the project's research goals.

In Roundsman, the five top-level attributes (see Table 5-1 page 83) are explicitly represented. Lower-level concerns (i.e., subattributes) however, are evaluated in an informal manner within procedures. For example, Roundsman explicitly represents the *cure* attribute, and may *procedurally* select ten-year results in preference to five-year results (subattributes). When evaluating this attribute another implementation might give five-year results a certain "weighting", ten-year results another weighting, etc. Roundsman simply uses the "preferred" ten-year data to evaluate the cure attribute. In order to acknowledge that additional data are relevant, Roundsman may parenthetically mention whether the additional data agree or disagree with the preferred data. (For example, in the critique excerpt shown on page 96, the preferred data are *recurrence-free* survival and the "other results" are data on *overall* survival.)

Roundsman's *procedural implementation* for evaluating the *subattributes* of the *cure* attribute can be divided into four steps. In steps 1 and 2 the relevant survival data are divided into two sets: "best" data and "additional" data. The "best" data are those data which are most highly preferred according to issues which are described under steps 1 and 2 below. The "additional" data are not discarded, but are carried through step 3 *in parallel* with the best data. Step 4 incorporates the effects of the distance metric upon the conclusions of step 3. The assessment of cure, then, is implemented in these four steps:

1. Filter the survival data to select the data with *longest follow-up*. This means, for example, that five-year results are preferred to three-year results.

2. If both recurrence-free survival and overall survival are available, use *recurrence-free results*. (The oncologist prefers these as indicators of cure.)

   At this point Roundsman has grouped the relevant data into two sets: "best" data and "additional" data. Step 3 is carried out on the "best" data and also for the "additional" data. The "best" data will be the basis of choice, but the oncologist feels that it is important for the system to inform the physician-user as to whether the "additional" data support or disagree with those conclusion(s). Accordingly, the critique shown at the beginning of this section (see page 96) mentions whether the additional data agree or not.

3. Examine the data concerning different interventions *without* consideration of the distance metric and see if one alternative is superior. This analysis involves using the difference between the survival proportions (DP) and the standard error of that difference (SE) as follows:

   - If the difference (DP) is greater than twice the standard error (SE) then Roundsman concludes that *on the basis of statistical results* one intervention is *better* than the other.
     Otherwise,

   - if DP plus SE is within 0.1 of 0 (i.e., little or no difference between proportions), Roundsman concludes that the two interventions are *equivalent.*
     Otherwise,

   - Roundsman concludes that the results are *indecisive.* (Neither intervention is clearly better, although they are probably not equivalent.)

4. Examine the effects of the distance metric assessments upon the conclusions of step 3. Roundsman's distance metric allows distance assessments to correct the bare statistical results (DP and SE) to account for mismatches between the physician's decision context (patient or plan) and the study. In the current implementation, rough units of correction are used. For example a "dp-change" whose value is "toward-zero-small" (see Fig. 3-8) means that the corrected estimate of DP is closer to zero than the bare statistical result is. In other words, the distance assessment "toward-zero-small" indicates that *after considering a particular case-specific feature* there is less difference between the two interventions than the bare statistical results would suggest. (Chapter 4 provides a more detailed discussion of how distance assessments are coupled with statistical results.)

   Since the underlying scale for DP is -1 to +1, the distance assessments could well accommodate correction factors which were oriented to Bayesian inference. For example, a correction factor of 0.7 might be a more "exact" statement of how much the reported DP value should be moved toward zero (DP_{new} = .7 * DP_{old}). This is one sense in which the distance metric is *independent* of the approach to comparing alternatives. If coarse units of measurement like "toward-zero-small" are thought to be too ad hoc, then more precise units might be used by a system-builder. Roundsman's current implementation uses *approximate* correction factors, but Roundsman's use of a distance metric is not in concept at odds with more normative approaches to evaluating choice.

In Roundsman's current approach, in addition to the factors mentioned above, when the number of serious mismatches and methodological weaknesses exceeds three, Roundsman concludes that the results *considered in this particular clinical context* are indecisive. On the other hand, if the number of serious distance problems is three or less, Roundsman concludes that the bare statistical results are not changed by the distance assessments. This current approach of tolerating only three serious mismatches before Roundsman concludes that decisive statistical results are indecisive for the physician's purposes is empirically derived and used as a first rough approximation. The criteria can be changed quite easily as Roundsman is developed further.

The effect of these four steps can be seen in Roundsman's critiques. For example, the critique paragraph shown at the beginning of this section (page 96) shows Roundsman discussing:

- The implication of the bare statistical results for the "best" data: in this case, recurrence-free survival,

- whether the "additional" data agree or disagree, and

- the implications of the "best" data *after consideration of the distance assessments*. In the example shown, distance assessments were so serious that seemingly *decisive* statistical results became *indecisive* in the context of the particular patient and plan. Roundsman's critique also makes it clear that the difficulties were in mismatches (patient and plan) rather than in the study's methodology. On the other hand, if methodology was the difficulty, then Roundsman's critique would be different - in order to make clear the basis for its analysis.

5.11. Summary

Four comparison strategies have been outlined for use in modeling medical management. These strategies are not heuristics, but *restricted versions* of a general approach (MADM) which may help better model choice and explanation within a given domain. This chapter emphasizes several other points:

- Use of each strategy may require strong assumptions about the nature of a domain.
- The operational definitions and assumptions are domain-independent.
- Previous AI programs in medical management, reinterpreted as examples of these strategies, are seen to contain common underlying structures. The seemingly ad hoc approaches of those programs use one or more of these four strategies to select a therapy choice and to explain that choice.
- A domain must be studied carefully to determine which strategies or combination of strategies might be appropriate.
- When the strategies are applicable, better, less complex explanations may be possible *because* the strategies entail stronger assumptions, i.e., more knowledge about the domain.

This chapter develops a general model of choice and explanation which could be used in a computational model of reasoning from the clinical literature. The implementation of this model in the Roundsman system was not as general as the model itself would allow: the implementation was limited to that combination of strategies which was useful for the breast cancer domain. Roundsman first compares alternatives by their promise to cure the patient. When two alternatives are equivalent with respect to cure, its critique suggests that the physician consider the trade-offs in cosmetic damage, local recurrence rate and the surgical trauma of the alternatives. In other domains, different features of the general model of choice and explanation might well play a more central role.

Chapter 6
Interactions Between Studies

As the Roundsman project evolved, it became increasingly clear that the issue of interaction between different studies was both clinically important and technically challenging. In the current Roundsman system, there is no representation of inter-study relationships. Although Roundsman does not currently deal with such interactions, I have devoted this chapter to setting down my current thoughts on the subject in an organized fashion. Thus, this chapter provides a preliminary skeleton upon which future research can build.

There are two settings in which interactions between studies play a prominent role. Section 6.1 outlines key issues for *updating* a knowledge-base that is organized around the use of clinical studies. Section 6.2 provides examples of how the results of different research reports may *conflict*, and suggests how inter-study knowledge may help illuminate and partially resolve such conflict(s).

6.1. Updating Roundsman Over Time

Although the current Roundsman system contains no representation for relationships *between* studies, encoding such relationships will be crucial to maintaining this type of knowledge base. Because medical knowledge is constantly evolving, expert clinicians maintain their knowledge of the field by "updating" with readings from the clinical literature. Knowledge from a new study often impacts their existing knowledge of previous studies, and *inter-study* relationships are established. Analogous inter-study relationships must be represented by knowledge-based systems if they are to be capable of updating. This section outlines key issues for updating a knowledge-base that is organized around the use of clinical studies, and provides concrete examples from the domain of breast cancer management. Thus, this section provides a preliminary skeleton upon which future research can build.

The Modular Approach to Updating

One approach to "updating" a system such as Roundsman is to add studies to the knowledge-base in a modular fashion. That is, the new study is first read and assessed by the expert. Following that assessment, the basic statistical results and expert's clinical assessment of the experiment are captured in the system's existing data structures. The new study is entered into the library (with no other modification of the system itself -- knowledge about other studies or any "inter-study" knowledge).

The current Roundsman system was constructed in essentially this manner. At the same time, it was acknowledged that this "modular" approach was somewhat unrealistic because earlier studies are often reassessed in light of subsequent study data. Consequently, in order to help investigate the problems of updating knowledge, the Roundsman knowledge-base was built chronologically. (Studies from the 1960's were entered into the knowledge base before studies from the 1970's and so forth; studies published in 1985 were entered last.) Although it was not possible to "blind" the expert oncologist to information which came from later studies, a conscious effort was made to analyze each study in light of the assumptions and research environment of the time period in which it was published. The collaborating oncologist was able to simulate this because he has been clinically involved in this field for decades and is acutely aware of how the background assumptions have changed.

Challenges to the Assumptions of Modularity

As the Roundsman knowledge-base was incrementally built, difficulties stemming from the modularity assumption were documented. Possible solutions were noted but not implemented in Roundsman, which instead focussed on how to tailor the interpretation of a single study in light of particular clinical contexts, not on the problem of updating knowledge over time. Issues uncovered in the course of this research include the following:

1. An influential study introduces novel patient-descriptors or interventions
2. Knowledge from recent studies defines more useful patient-strata
3. A new study answers question(s) raised by a previous study
4. A new publication is based upon an ongoing study with prior publications
5. New research report suggests a special, sweeping reinterpretation of previous report

The remainder of this section discusses particular examples of these changes, and outlines the challenges they pose for knowledge base management.

1. An influential study introduces novel patient-descriptors or interventions

Clinical investigators may use an unusual technique that is not the focus of the study per se, but is a standard component of the study design. Often it is a subjective judgment as to whether the technique in question is essential to achieving the results reported. (It may require further research to determine that. For an nice illustration of this, see the oncology example provided below under issue #3 .) At the very least, a critical appraisal should mention that this unusual technique was employed. If the study is influential, the new technique will become an important entity in the field, and will have an impact upon the interpretation of prior and subsequent clinical studies.

Example from Oncology Management: The NSABP-06 trial [Fisher 85a], identified in the Roundsman library as Fisher85a, investigated "verified wide excision". (Excision, sometimes called "lumpectomy", is one surgical approach to the management of primary breast cancer. Excision removes only the tumor, leaving as much breast tissue as possible.) Excision of tumor was not a new intervention (earlier empirical investigations had studied it as well) but Fisher's protocol specified that before a woman was entered into the "verified wide excision" arm of the study, the excised tissue must have been examined by a pathologist who *verified* that the specimen margins did not contain tumor. This assured that the population of women studied had small tumor dimensions. (Size estimates from physical exam may be inaccurate, and the "verified wide excision" process screens out women with deceptively large tumors.) One effect of Fisher85a has been to inject new vocabulary into breast cancer management: *verified* wide excision. Prior to the NSABP-06 trial, clinical studies rarely reported whether the specimen margins contained tumor. The publication of Fisher85a in March of 1985 has had the effect of encouraging the inclusion of this information in pathology reports, and most oncologists now want to know about excision margins before they suggest therapy.

As mentioned above, the Roundsman system was built incrementally and studies were added in chronological order. When an influential study introduced novel patient-descriptors or interventions, new data structures (e.g., a new type of treatment) were defined for the system. Subsequent additions to the knowledge-base of studies were then able to use those new data structures. This solution is suboptimal because the system cannot intelligently assess the relationships *between* the older studies and studies using the newer definitions. A more general solution must be sought for this issue which arises repeatedly as medical knowledge evolves.

2. Knowledge from recent studies defines more useful patient-strata

Research reports may demonstrate that intervention-A is superior to intervention-B, *but only for certain patient types.* Previous studies may have found no difference between two interventions when they examined coarser strata of patients. (The patients who might be responsive to treatment A were lost in a larger set of unresponsive patients.) Identification of more precise patient-strata may well force a reinterpretation of the study's "no difference" conclusion. The identification of more precise patient strata may also allow one to estimate how the results of a prior study might change if its protocol were altered slightly. (Of course, this kind of subjective extrapolation is not without danger.)

Example from Oncology Management: Studies on chemotherapeutic treatment of primary breast cancer were suggesting by about 1983 that chemotherapy improved survival for *pre-menopausal* women. Prior studies which did not stratify by menopausal status might easily have concluded that chemotherapy offered no advantages to women with breast cancer. After 1983, it might be reasonable to say that for a pre-menopausal patient we could achieve results which are superior to a study which did *not* include chemotherapy as part of its protocol (e.g., surgery alone).

The current Roundsman system does accommodate this type of updating. The system maintainer can create additional instances of a data structure called the *distance-estimator* [Rennels 86b]. Distance-estimators allow the Roundsman system to assess various "distances" between the conditions of the clinical study (e.g., patient population, protocol followed, etc.) and the conditions which the physician faces (e.g., specific patient and current treatment plan). Thus, entry of a new study into Roundsman's knowledge base might entail the creation of a new *distance-estimator* which would then in turn operate on existing studies when appropriate.

3. A new study answers question(s) raised by a previous study

When a promising therapy emerges, clinicians may not know whether *all* components of the protocol used in the published study contribute to the favorable end results. It may be impossible to confidently omit a particular component without some concern that the patient will suffer harm. If a subsequent study isolates that component as the subject of investigation, the results may allow a more thorough understanding of the contribution each component made to the results seen in the prior study. It would be important for a system providing advice from the clinical literature to encode the interrelationships between this recent clinical report and those previous studies which are now somewhat better understood.

Example from Oncology Management: In the 1960's and 1970's there was a good deal of encouraging experimental data concerning the use of total mastectomy in combination with adjuvant radiotherapy. (Total mastectomy is a surgical procedure in which all breast tissue is removed.) It was not known what portion of the observed effect was due to the radiation. In the absence of experimental data, expert opinion held that dropping the radiation would lower the survival somewhat. Fisher80 [Fisher 80] contributed solid evidence that adjuvant radiation had no effect on survival when the surgical approach was total mastectomy. That is, the expert consensus was actually incorrect, and was overturned only after an appropriate body of experimental evidence [Fisher 80] became available. This new study supersedes the expert opinion mentioned earlier, rendering it somewhat *obsolete*. Fisher80 is thus quite important since it alters the interpretation of earlier studies.

In the current Roundsman system, this interaction is handled by *modifying* the appropriate distance-estimator. Interpretation of the earlier studies is performed by the modified distance-estimator, formerly based only on an expert's clinical assessment, but now based on the experimental evidence in Fisher80.

4. A new publication is based upon an ongoing study with prior publications

Publishing new results from the same basic study might be viewed as simply "wiping out old knowledge". Yet the manner in which clinicians reason from clinical literature makes it advantageous for a knowledge-based system to retain the previous publication and to represent *explicitly* the relationship between the new and old study. In many cases it would be useful for the system to have specific knowledge of the relative strengths and weaknesses of closely related studies.

Example from Oncology Management: Peters77 [Peters 77] updates Peters67 [Peters 67]. Peters77 not only provides longer follow-up than Peters67 but also improves upon the experimental design of Peters67 by "matching" patients according to age, year of treatment, and tumor size. If the physician user, unaware of Peters77, cited Peters67 as support for his reasoning it would be important for the system to display knowledge of Peters67 (not possible if updating involved "wiping out" the old study) and to argue for use of Peters77 because it provides matching of controls as well as longer follow-up.

The Roundsman system encodes linkages between publications from the same (ongoing) study, and Roundsman simply discusses the most recent of the publications. (The system can be run for any year between 1950 and 1985. The critiques generated differ depending on the year specified.) Roundsman has little or no information on why the most recent study is preferred. A cleaner and more general solution would include a knowledge representation for those preferences.

5. New research report suggests a special, sweeping reinterpretation of previous report

In some situations the insight gained by a new biomedical report is unique and does not fall neatly into any of the categories enumerated above. The most appropriate way for a knowledge-based system to incorporate such new knowledge might be simply to allow modification of the *explanatory* material stored with previous studies in the system's knowledge-base.

Example from Oncology Management: Interpretation of the NSABP-06 trial [Fisher 85a] was somewhat difficult because the effect of verifying that excision margins were free of tumor was not entirely clear. Did margin verification affect the results and if so, how? Subsequent publications [Recht 85, E. Fisher 86], although weak methodologically, suggest that the women who do poorly with excision (compared to mastectomy) might be those with *multifocal* tumor. At this point, one might view the NSABP-06 trial [Fisher 85a] in a new light. Perhaps *verification* screens out multifocal tumors (numerous foci would presumably cause more of the specimens to have tumor in the excision margins) and thus excludes those women most likely to do poorly with excision. In other words, although the purpose of verification was to exclude *large* tumors, it may well have also screened out women with *multifocal* tumors.

In the Roundsman project, sweeping reinterpretations of previous reports were handled in a case-by-case fashion, and no general solution was implemented. Our experience with this problem suggests, however, that the updating of systems like Roundsman provides an excellent laboratory to probe the difficulties and the potential rewards of knowledge-representation research.

6.2. Conflict Between Study Results

This section discusses approaches to combining results of more than one study, especially when their research results are in conflict. Roundsman currently adjusts only for the mismatches between a single study and the decision context (as described in Chapter 4). A further goal (not currently implemented) would be to assess the *combined* implications of more than one study. Two examples of conflict in such settings are introduced (below) and discussed more fully later in the section.

Example 1: Excision (Lumpectomy) for Stage II Breast Cancer

The results of the Guy's hospital trial [Atkins 72, Hayward 77] suggest that wide excision with adjuvant radiotherapy is *unsafe* (compared to mastectomy) for stage II patients. (Indeed, the investigators of the Guy's trial stopped randomizing stage II patients because they felt it was unethical to give women wide excision when experimental results indicated it endangered their lives.) The experimental results were not as clear for stage I patients but a *subsequent* trial at Guy's hospital [Hayward 83] studied stage I patients and *also* found that excision with adjuvant radiotherapy was *unsafe* (compared to mastectomy). The results of the NSABP-06 study [Fisher 85a], published in March of 1985, suggest that wide excision and adjuvant radiotherapy is *safe* for women with stage I *and* stage II breast cancer, implying that such women do *not* require a mastectomy.

Example 2: Postmenopausal Estrogen Use and Heart Disease

Two research reports on the relationship between postmenopausal estrogen use and heart disease were published in the same issue of *The New England Journal of Medicine* [Wilson 85, Stampfer 85]. The publication by Stampfer et al. concludes that postmenopausal hormones protect women against heart disease, resulting in a relative risk of 0.30 for coronary disease among current users of estrogens and 0.59 among past users. The other publication, by Wilson et al., is a report from the Framingham study, a highly reputable epidemiological research project concerning heart disease. They studied virtually the same question as Stampfer et al. and concluded that postmenopausal hormones substantially *increases* the risk of cardiovascular disease: among a mixed group of current and past users the relative risk was 1.90.

Clearly, studies that compare treatments do not always agree with each other. Should a system such as Roundsman point out the controversy and disclaim responsibility for any final *combined* estimate? *Can* the results be combined? This section discusses two general approaches to the problem: (1) Bayes' Estimation and Meta-Analysis, and (2) explicit use of expert "supra-study" knowledge.

6.2.1. Bayes' Estimates and Meta-Analysis

What are the possibilities for using Bayes' rule to estimate the combined results? Since studies are usually published over a period of years, it seems quite natural to update *prior* knowledge based on study-1 with new information coming from study-2 in order to arrive at a *posterior* estimate for the parameter of interest. Unfortunately, Bayes' estimation is not always appropriate for this situation. The observations made below about the form of Bayes' estimates are not novel: they can be found in standard textbooks of statistics. (For example, see the discussion of conjugate families in [Lindgren 76].) The purpose of the following exposition is to consider whether Bayes' estimation is a reasonable approach to combining the evidence from two clinical studies.

In Roundsman, it is of interest to find an estimate of the *difference between proportions*, abbreviated below as "DP". The value of DP lies between -1.0 and +1.0.. The density function of interest is the probability of DP given the evidence from more than one clinical study. This density function is denoted as $P(DP \mid CS_1, CS_2)$. (Clinical study$_i$ is written "CS_i".) It is assumed that $P(DP \mid CS_1)$ and $P(DP \mid CS_2)$ can be determined by analyzing the relevance of each study to the given clinical context. CS_i stands for a complex set of evidence: it includes the proportions observed (p_1 and p_2), the statistical design, the sample size, and adjustment(s) for population mismatches or intervention mismatches.

Without any prior information there is no reason to believe that DP equals any one particular value within -1.0 to 1.0 more than any other particular value. That is, P(DP) is a uniform distribution. Since P(DP) is a constant, $P(DP \mid CS_i)$ can be rearranged:

$$P(DP \mid CS_i)$$

$$= P(CS_i \mid DP)\, P(DP) \;/\; \int_{DP} P(CS_i \mid DP) P(DP)$$

$$= k \cdot P(CS_i \mid DP) \tag{1}$$

where k is a normalization constant.

This rearrangement indicates that if the prior is a uniform distribution, then updating with new information gives back the same functional form as the prior (except that it must be re-normalized in order to have area = 1).

In the set of equalities below, $P(DP \mid CS_1, CS_2)$ is shown to equal an expression which is solvable.

$$P(DP \mid CS_1, CS_2)$$

$$= k' \cdot P(CS_1, CS_2 \mid DP)\, P(DP) \tag{2}$$

by Bayes' theorem,
where k' is a normalization constant.

$$= k' \cdot k'' \cdot P(CS_1, CS_2 \mid DP)$$

since P(DP) is a constant.

$$= k' \cdot k'' \cdot P(CS_1 \mid DP)\, P(CS_2 \mid DP)$$

by the assumed conditional independence of studies,
i.e., that $P(CS_1 \mid DP, CS_2) = P(CS_1 \mid DP)$.

$$= k' \cdot k'' \cdot k''' \cdot k'''' \cdot P(DP \mid CS_1)\, P(DP \mid CS_2) \tag{3}$$

by 1.

As mentioned above, $P(DP \mid CS_i)$ is assumed known from Roundsman's assessment of $study_i$ in the context of a patient and a proposed intervention. Consequently 3 is the algebraic product of known distributions (modified by normalization constants).

The density function for DP is assumed to have a normal, or gaussian form (approximating a binomial)[5]. How is the mean and variance of the *product* of two normal distributions related to the mean and variance of the two starting distributions which were multiplied together? The probability density function for the normal distribution is $f(x) = (1/\sqrt{2\pi\sigma})\cdot\exp[-(x-\mu)^2/2\sigma^2]$. Multiplying together the functions for the two normal distributions $N(\mu_1, \sigma_1^2)$ and $N(\mu_2, \sigma_2^2)$ yields a coefficient (which I disregard for the moment) and an exponent. By examining the form of the resulting exponent it is possible to write the mean and variance of the resulting distribution in terms of μ_1, σ_1, μ_2 and σ_2.

The exponent (of the product)

$$= -(x^2-2x\mu_1+\mu_1^2)/2\sigma_1^2 \; - \; (x^2-2x\mu_2+\mu_2^2)/2\sigma_2^2.$$

Multiplying to obtain a common denominator,

$$= [-2\sigma_2^2x^2 + 2\sigma_2^2 2x\mu_1 - 2\sigma_2^2\mu_1^2 - 2\sigma_1^2x^2 + 2\sigma_1^2 2x\mu_2 - 2\sigma_1^2\mu_2^2] \;/\; 4\sigma_1^2\sigma_2^2$$

collecting terms in the numerator,

$$= [x^2(\sigma_1^2+\sigma_2^2)(-2) - 2x(\sigma_2^2\mu_1 + \sigma_1^2\mu_2)(-2) + (\sigma_2^2\mu_1^2 + \sigma_1^2\mu_2^2)(-2)] \;/\; 4\sigma_1^2\sigma_2^2$$

factoring out $(\sigma_1^2 + \sigma_2^2)(-2)$,

$$= (\sigma_1^2+\sigma_2^2)(-2)\,[x^2 - 2x(\sigma_2^2\mu_1+\sigma_1^2\mu_2)/(\sigma_1^2+\sigma_2^2) + (\sigma_2^2\mu_1^2+\sigma_1^2\mu_2^2)/(\sigma_1^2+\sigma_2^2)] \;/\; 4\sigma_1^2\sigma_2^2$$

dividing numerator and denominator by $2(\sigma_1^2+\sigma_2^2)$,

$$= -[x^2 - 2x(\sigma_2^2\mu_1 + \sigma_1^2\mu_2)/(\sigma_1^2+\sigma_2^2) + C] \;/\; 2[\sigma_1\sigma_2/\sqrt{(\sigma_1^2+\sigma_2^2)}\,]^2. \quad (4)$$

The leftover constant C is expected because the resulting distribution must be re-normalized. Exponent 4 fits a normal distribution whose exponent is $(x-\mu_3)^2/2\sigma_3^2$,

---

[5]For values of DP reasonably close to zero and a moderate standard error, the normal approximation is a good one. This approximation will break down as the effects of the two procedures get more different. In this case, beta distributions might be a better family of density functions to use than the normal distribution. It is important to note however, that the principal issue here -- the narrowing of the standard deviation with additional studies -- would *also* apply to beta distributions. The difficult question is unchanged: Are the two experiments studying precisely the same question (i.e., parameters) or is there some difference along undetected parameter(s) that is responsible for the disagreement? In the latter case it is misleading to "update" with Bayes' formula.

where

$$\mu_3 = (\sigma_2^2\mu_1 + \sigma_1^2\mu_2)/(\sigma_1^2+\sigma_2^2), \quad \text{and} \tag{5}$$

$$\sigma_3 = \sigma_1\sigma_2 \;/\; \sqrt{(\sigma_1^2+\sigma_2^2)}. \tag{6}$$

From 5 it can be seen that the posterior mean is a weighted average of μ_1 and μ_2. Recall the two studies of postmenopausal estrogen use and heart disease. The Bayes' estimate of the mean might be approximately 0. If we had to make a point estimate for μ, the Bayes' estimate might suffice.

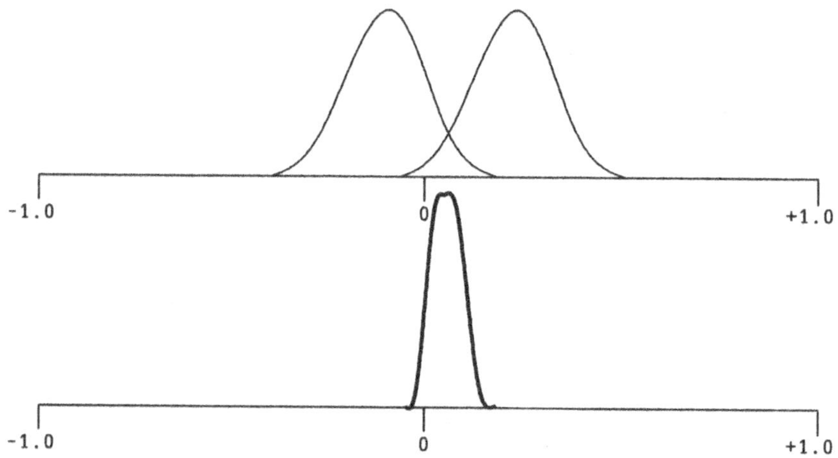

Figure 6-1: Bayesian updating.
The prior distribution (top right) is updated with new information (top left). The posterior distribution (bottom figure) has a mean that is a weighted average of the other two, and a variance that is *smaller* than the variance of either the prior or the new information.

For the purposes of combining studies whose results disagree, the problem with Bayes' estimation[6] lies in the posterior variance. A slight rearrangement of 6 shows

---

[6]Standard statistical notation might describe Bayesian updating somewhat differently than I have done. One might restate the problem as follows: Assume that one is estimating a parameter X which is drawn from a normal distribution of mean μ and variance σ^2, denoted $X \sim N(\mu, \sigma^2)$. The first study provides *prior* information, specifically that $\mu \sim N(\nu, \tau^2)$. Then in the second study we observe X=x. What is the *posterior* distribution for μ? The posterior mean is $(x\tau^2 + \nu\sigma^2)/(\sigma^2+\tau^2)$. The posterior variance is $(\sigma^2\tau^2)/(\sigma^2 + \tau^2)$.

that $\sigma_3 = \sigma_1 (\sigma_2 / \sqrt{(\sigma_1^2+\sigma_2^2)})$. That is, σ_3 is *smaller* than either σ_1 or σ_2. This relationship is depicted in Fig. 6-1.

Example 2 revisited: Postmenopausal Estrogen Use and Heart Disease

Consider again the two studies on use of postmenopausal estrogens. Aside from gross errors, what could produce such conflicting results? The experienced clinician or biostatistician might conjecture that there is "more than one answer". That is, the two studies are measuring different things. There is at least one more "degree of freedom" to these data than was used to analyze it.

It is possible to identify differences between the two studies: in one study the subjects were nurses, while in the other study the subjects were women from various job descriptions. One study mailed questionnaires while the other study conducted interviews. The definition of menopause differed somewhat between the two groups, as did the precise type of estrogen used and the dosages. But do those details makes clear the reason for such a tremendous conflict in conclusions? The expert referees who reviewed the paper were unable to say what might explain the conflict. In an editorial accompanying these two papers, biostatistician and physician John Bailar states,

> "I simply cannot tell from present evidence whether these hormones add to the risk of various cardiovascular diseases, diminish the risk, or leave it unchanged, and must resort to the investigator's great cop-out: More research is needed." [Bailar 85]

When patients ask for advice, however, physicians do not have the luxury of postponing recommendations until this question is investigated with subsequent studies. An answer of some sort must be forthcoming.

With regard to these two publications on estrogen and heart disease, one study tells us that estrogens increase the risk of heart disease, and the other tells us that estrogens decrease the risk. How well does the Bayes' updating procedure serve us in this situation? Recall that the combined variance is smaller than either of the two separate variances. Is it reasonable that the *combined* estimate of risk should have a smaller variance (*less* uncertainty about the truth) than either of the two *separate* studies? Faced with these two conflicting bodies of evidence, the clinician might well be *more* uncertain about the true value than he would be if only one of the studies had been published.

In this situation, an argument might be made for a rule of combination that *adds* the two distributions, as shown in Fig. 6-2. This would leave intact the sense of there being controversy and great uncertainty as to the truth, yet allow one to look at a composite result in order to make decisions.

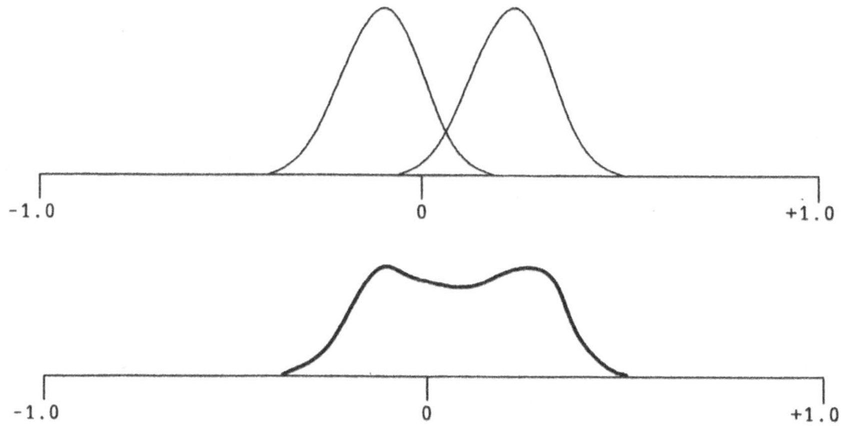

Figure 6-2: Schematic of an averaging process.
The prior (top right) and the new information (top left) are averaged to produce a posterior distribution (bottom figure). The mean of the posterior is a weighted average of the other two, but a variance that is *larger* than the variance of either the prior or the new information.

<u>**Meta-Analysis:**</u> Combining the results of more than one study is an extremely active area of research in biostatistics. It is often referred to as "meta-analysis". Some published work, for example [Halvorsen 83], discuss various approaches to determining a reasonable *combined* estimate for the value of a parameter. Very little of that work, however, concerns how to arrive at a posterior estimate of the uncertainty (standard error) of that combined estimate.

A recent example of meta-analysis is work by Dr. Peto (unpublished)[7] that was important testimony in the National Consensus Panel Meeting on the Use of Adjuvant Chemotherapy for Breast Cancer which took place in September, 1985. Dr. Peto tackled one of the most vexing problems of current breast cancer therapy: the numerous and conflicting reports on the effectiveness of the drug tamoxifen for women with breast cancer. Dr. Peto analyzed the *raw data* from a large number of published *and* unpublished studies, and subsequently combined the data into larger

---

[7]This work may remain unpublished because some of the investigators who provided the primary data have not given permission for publication of the analytical results based on their data.

sets -- essentially creating a study with larger sample sizes. His analysis is not without controversy: some of the people who provided data to him disagree with his approach to analyzing it. To illustrate the difficulties of meta-analysis, let us suppose that Dr. Peto looked at data from studies in which one group of women were treated with PF (i.e., the chemotherapeutic agents L-PAM and 5-FU) and another group received PFT (L-PAM, 5-FU *and* tamoxifen). For purposes of analysis, Dr. Peto might then *factor out* the PF and consider these trials to be studies of placebo versus tamoxifen. If this assumption can be made then the results from these studies can be *pooled* with those of studies which *actually* studied placebo versus tamoxifen. One problem with this assumption is that the effect of PF and tamoxifen are not independent: tamoxifen has been shown (in the lab) to affect the cellular uptake of chemotherapy. Dr. Peto's work is one basis for the recommendations of the National Consensus Panel Meeting. It illustrates the importance of meta-analysis in reasoning from experimental evidence.

The meta-analysis problem is in the critical path of modeling the process of reasoning from the clinical literature. It is a non-trivial problem that does not seem, at present, to be solvable by any numerical approach alone. I expect that for the foreseeable future, useful analysis of multiple studies will draw heavily upon explicit knowledge of the domain of application, as exhibited in the discussion of Dr. Peto's work (above). Meta-analysis decisions will depend on a good deal of subjective judgment. This, in turn, means that a decision support system such as Roundsman must explicitly represent a significant amount of inter-study domain knowledge.

6.2.2. Explicit Use of Inter-Study Domain Knowledge

The statistical approaches outlined above try to combine the studies primarily on a numerical basis. A much more clinically useful approach might be to use *explicit expert knowledge* about the relationships between studies, i.e., "supra-study" knowledge. Resolving conflicts via a strictly numerical approach is extremely difficult and not as clinically illuminating as using the domain expert's clinical judgment about inter-study relationships.

Example 1 Revisited: Excision (Lumpectomy) for Stage II Breast Cancer

As described earlier in this chapter, there is outstanding conflict between results from the Guy's Hospital trial [Atkins 72, Hayward 77, Hayward 83], which suggests that excision plus radiation of breast cancer is unsafe, and other trials [Veronesi 81, Amalric 82, Fisher 85a] which suggest that excision plus radiation is safe. The most common *explanation* for the conflicting results is that the radiation dosages used in the Guy's Hospital trial were too low, but this remains a matter of some speculation. Nevertheless, as the tenor of the field has changed and radiation dose standards have settled at levels higher than the Guy's Hospital dose, the Guy's trial has become more remote from the clincal decision about breast cancer surgery. In the minds of many physicians, the conflict is side-stepped by choosing to pay attention only to the trials which used higher dosages. That is, in this case a *domain-specific assumption* is crucial to the practitioner's resolution of conflicting results.

Because the questions surrounding the Guy's Hospital trial are not entirely answered, new interpretations (aside from radiation dose) arise. As discussed earlier in this chapter, studies by [Recht 85] and [E. Fisher 86] (although weak methodologically) suggest that women with *multifocal* tumor do more poorly with excision than mastectomy. This explicit domain knowledge may explain the conflicting results of the Guy's Hospital trial and the NSABP trial. Verification of tumor-free margins would screen out multifocal tumors and thus excludes those women most likely to do poorly without mastectomy. Since the Guy's trial did not require *verified* wide excision, the inferior results of excision in the Guy's trial might be secondary to including a sizeable group of women with multifocal tumors. Again, a domain-specific judgment is central to this interpretation of conflicting results.

The expert oncologist makes clinical judgments of this sort when evaluating the experimental evidence contained in the papers published in his field. By explicitly representing this information, Roundsman might be capable of shedding light upon certain conflicts which are not well handled solely by techniques of numerical combination.

6.3. Summary and Future Directions

Future knowledge-based systems may well provide a sophisticated analysis of the clinical literature for physicians who are considering a particular patient and treatment plan. Augmenting these systems with a newly published study would ideally accomplish what human experts do when "updating" their knowledge of the field (reading and assessing new biomedical reports). This chapter has outlined certain key issues for accomplishing this updating process and has provided examples of these issues from the oncology literature. As illustrated in the examples, adding new studies should involve much more than "filling in slots" of a pre-determined representation scheme. The unique characteristics of a research report often cast previous reports in a new light, altering their interpretation. A promising direction for future research is the development of sophisticated approaches to update automatically the knowledge-base of systems based on the clinical literature. This would entail automatically assisting the user in entering a new study. Central to this process would be mechanisms to help the user encode the *inter-study* relationships that arise.

Explicit encoding of expert knowledge about inter-study relationships might not only assist numerical approaches such as meta-analysis but might also offer different approaches. For example, when a new study is entered the system might scan the studies already in its knowledge base, attempt to anticipate conflicts, and then ask the person entering the study how such conflicts should be handled. In its critique Roundsman might "factor out" the confounding issues. That is, it might offer its observations prefaced with commentary that the analysis is deliberately ignoring certain issues (e.g., the interaction of tamoxifen with cellular uptake of chemotherapy). Alternatively, Roundsman might explicitly identify the troublesome issues (e.g., presence or absence of tumor-free excision margins) and ask the user which study fits the user's clinical situation most closely. It might then preferentially use one study, ignoring the other study. It is anticipated that the development of a knowledge updating facility would be a vehicle to explore and clarify many additional aspects of reasoning from the empirical evidence in clinical literature.

In summary, it is clear that the related problems of updating knowledge and dealing with the interactions between studies offer a fertile area for future research. This chapter has attempted to expose some of the basic issues upon which this research can build.

Chapter 7
Text Generation

Object-Oriented Text Generation from an Expert System

7.1. Introduction

Text generation is an extremely valuable adjunct to expert system advisors: the advice becomes accessible to a wider audience. Examples of successful use of explanation and text generation facilities within an expert system include MYCIN's translator [Buchanan 84] and ATTENDING's use of PROSENET [Miller 84]. Expert system builders may often feel they cannot afford to develop their own text generation program. Research issues which are more central to their projects may take priority.

This section describes a straightforward, relatively easily implemented approach to text generation for an expert system. The design is called TEXTNET, adapted for Roundsman from PROSENET [Miller 84] but recast in the object-oriented paradigm [Stefik 86]. This chapter describes the TEXTNET data structures in terms *generic* to object-oriented programming so that it is clear exactly what is required to build and use the TEXTNET approach in any object-oriented programming language.

TEXTNET is based on the notion of "augmented transition networks" (ATNs), originally devloped for natural language analysis [Woods 70, Miller 74]. ATNs consist of *states* and of *arcs* which connect the states. These ATNs are "traversed" by moving from state to state across arcs. TEXTNET can be viewed as a collection of individual ATN's. In this description each separate ATN is referred to as a *net*. The system builder constructs each net with an eye toward its eventual integration into an overall collection of nets, for example, a hierarchy of nets.

Each net is designed to express (in prose form) some information which the system-builder wants to communicate to the user. A sample TEXTNET net is shown in Fig. 7-1. States are depicted as circles labelled with letters. Arcs are depicted as arrows connecting the states. All states are shown as circles in this schematic, but TEXTNET states are not all alike. A state is one of five types:

1. Start-State: (e.g., "start-state-net-1" in Fig. 7-1). There is one Start-State per net. Processing of a net begins on the Start-State.

2. Pop-State: (e.g., state N in Fig. 7-1). Processing of a net terminates on the Pop-State.

3. Cond-State: (e.g., states B, D and M in Fig. 7-1). A Cond-State *cond*itionally chooses one of the arcs leading away from itself by assessing certain local information.

4. Option-State: (e.g., state E in Fig. 7-1). An Option-State *randomly* chooses one of its arcs.

5. Sequence-State: (e.g., state H in Fig. 7-1). A Sequence-State chooses one of its arcs according to that arc's position in a specified sequence.

Traversal of an arc results in a side effect, for example sending text to a printer buffer. Arcs are one of five types:

1. Text-Arc: (e.g., the arcs between states B and C in Fig. 7-1). Traversal of a Text-Arc causes a pre-stored text string to be sent to the printer buffer.

2. Function-Arc: (e.g., the arcs between states C and D in Fig. 7-1). Traversal of a Function-Arc causes the evaluation of a procedure defined by the system-builder. The value returned from that procedure is then sent to the printer buffer.

3. Jump-Arc: (e.g., the top arc between states G and I in Fig. 7-1). Traversal of this arc results in immediate traversal to the next state, without side effects. These arcs are used to bypass text which need not be output in certain situations. Examples of the use of jump-arcs are provided below.

4. Push-Arc: e.g., the arc between states I and M in Fig. 7-1. When a Push-Arc is traversed, the system "pushes" down to a lower net, and temporarily suspends processing of the net in which this Push-Arc is located. When the Pop-State of the lower net is encountered, the system "pops" back up to this Push-Arc and continues.

5. Endsequence-Arc: e.g., the lower arc between states M and H in Fig. 7-1. The Endsequence-Arc has a very specific purpose. It's sole use is to

signal a Sequence-State to reinitialize itself when there are no more items in the sequence it is currently processing.

7.2. Examples

This section describes how the states and arcs of Fig. 7-1 are used, and gives sample output from traversal of this net. Each net has available to it certain information which it uses to determine which arcs to traverse. The net shown in Fig. 7-1 is designed to make comments about clinical studies. Consequently, this net has access to a local variable, "study-list", which is a list of studies.

Processing begins on the start state ("start-state-net-1" in Fig. 7-1) and automatically moves to state A, which is a Cond-State. Cond-State A has only one arc, so that Text-Arc is traversed, sending the text string "there" to the printer buffer. Cond-State B examines study-list, determines that its length is greater than 1, and chooses the top Text-Arc, sending the string "are" to the printer buffer. Cond-State C has only one arc, a Function-Arc which determines the length of study-list and then sends that integer to the printer buffer.

Cond-State D chooses the top arc (for the same reason state B chose its top arc) causing the string "studies" to be sent to the printer buffer. Option-State E randomly chooses the Text-Arc "pertinent to this patient", causing that string to be sent to the printer buffer. The sole arc between states F and J is traversed, sending the "*period" punctuation symbol to the printer buffer. Similarly, the arc between states J and G sends a "*para" (new paragraph) punctuation symbol to the printer.

Cond-State G examines the length of study-list and because the length is greater than 1 it chooses the bottom arc to state H, a Jump-Arc which causes no side effect except progressing to state H. Sequence-State H chooses the first arc in its sequence of arcs, sending the string "first," to the printer buffer. Cond-State I chooses its only arc, the Push-Arc between I and M. This arc causes the system to "push" down to net-2, which coordinates discussion of one clinical study. When the system completes processing of net-2 it "pops" back up to proceed to state M.

Cond-State M takes the front study off study-list and examines the length of the new study-list. Since there are more studies to discuss, it chooses the top arc (*para) between state M and state H. This Text-Arc sends a *para punctuation symbol to the printer buffer. State H then chooses the second arc in the series, causing the string "second" to be sent to the printer buffer. Eventually, state M finds that study-list is empty, and chooses the bottom Endsequence-Arc back to state H. Finally, the Jump-Arc between state H and the Pop-State N terminates processing of net-1.

Sample output from processing of net-1 is shown below. The prose generated by

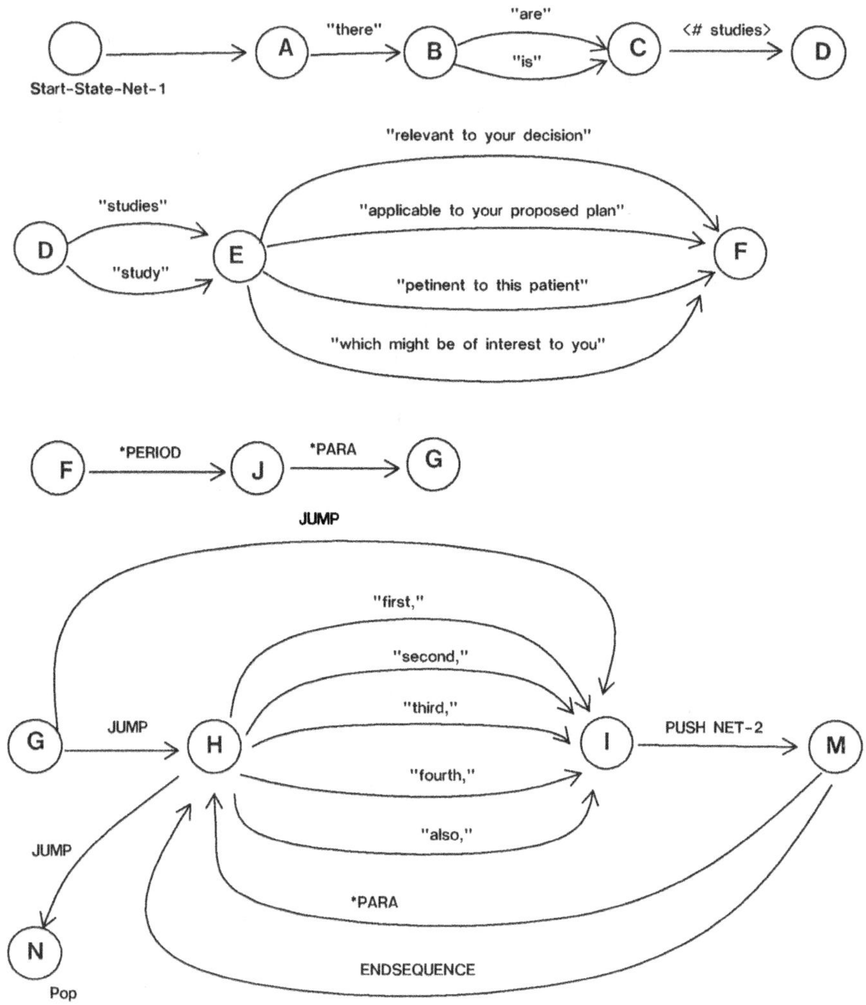

Figure 7-1: Sample net, called "Net-1".

lower nets is replaced by bracketed notation of these lower nets.

"There are 2 studies pertinent to this patient.

"First, ... <push to net-2>

"Second, ... <push to net-2>

As was mentioned earlier, during the processing of net-1, the system pushes down to net-2. A schematic representation of net-2 is shown in Fig. 7-2. The sample prose shown below includes the output from net-2. As before, the prose from lower nets has been edited out, and replaced with bracketed notation indicating the name of the net.

"There are 2 studies pertinent to this patient.

"First, Peters77 employed non-randomized controls in a study performed by investigators at Princess Margaret Hospital, Toronto. <push to net-4> ... <push to net-6>

"Second, Atkins72 was a randomized, controlled trial carried out at Guy's Hospital, England. <push to net-3>...<push to net-6>

The third sample of prose output (below) shows the text generated when four levels of nets are included. This is an example from the Roundsman system.

"There are 2 studies pertinent to this patient.

"First, Peters77 employed non-randomized controls in a study performed by investigators at Princess Margaret Hospital, Toronto. A set of patients who were treated by wide excision combined with adjuvant radiotherapy (203) is compared against treatment with radical mastectomy combined with adjuvant radiotherapy (609). For patients who underwent the first protocol the recurrence-free survival at five years turned out to be 0.7, recurrence-free survival at ten years was equal to 0.6, overall survival at five years was 0.85 and overall survival at ten years was equal to 0.75. In the group which received the second protocol the recurrence-free survival at five years was 0.7, recurrence-free survival at ten years was 0.6, overall survival at five years was 0.8 and overall survival at ten years was 0.68.

"How do these data apply to your patient? We are not particularly concerned that the intervention was somewhat nonstandard (about 10% of each group didn't get the radiotherapy). More troublesome is that the study population was probably in a better prognostic stratum than your

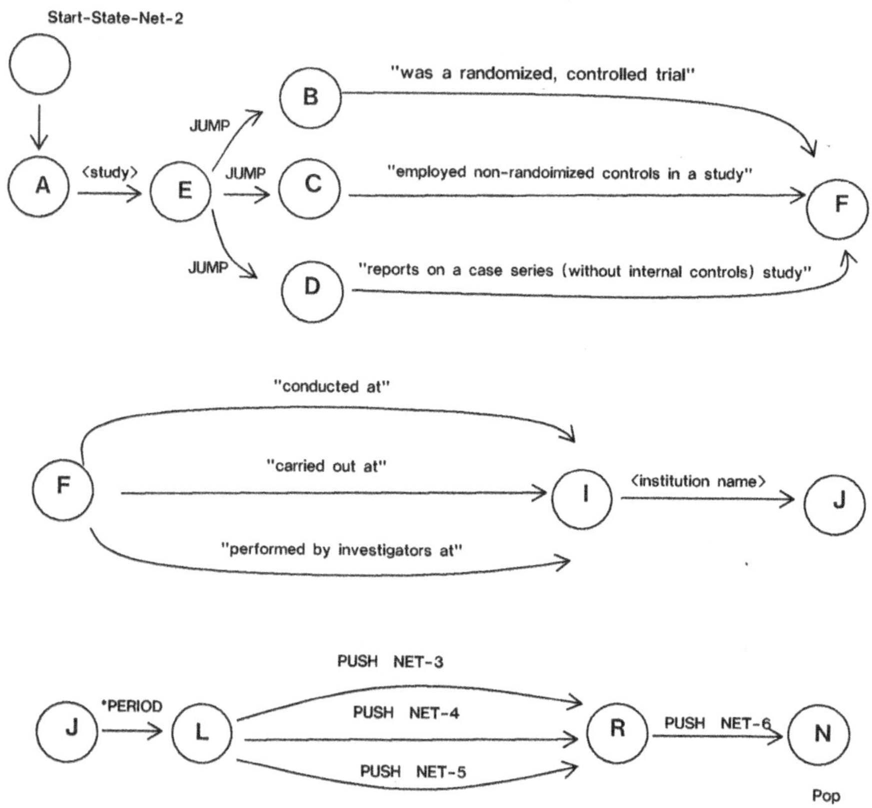

Figure 7-2: A sample net, called "Net-2".

patient (they were clinically node negative).

"Reviewing the study itself, the results are weakened because first, statistical reporting was sketchy (data reported as graphs without P values or standard errors). Second, we suspect that a selection bias was introduccd (e.g., tumor size assessed by same physicians who chose treatment). Third, choice of treatment was decided non-randomly (although Peters did match controls for T size, age & treatment year). Fourth, patients were accrued over a rather long period (patient entry lasted from 1939 to 1972). "

" Second, Atkins72 was a randomized, controlled trial ... <etc.>

7.3. Programming Language Primitives: Objects and Messages

As mentioned previously, the TEXTNET approach may be adapted easily to any object-oriented environment. The underlying programming language is assumed to have 1) objects, and 2) messages which can be received by those objects. Objects are abstract data types, usually thought of as frame-based, containing slots for storing various features of the objects. The declaration of an object involves specifying its particular set of slots and messages. The programmer must declare what action is to be taken when each possible message is received. In essence, messages (which may have arguments) are procedures stored with the object upon which they operate. In a TEXTNET, states are represented as objects with arcs stored in slots. The messages of a state help determine which arc will be traversed next. The messages of an arc help determine the effect of traversing that arc.

For example, TEXTNET's Option-State object has one slot, Arc-Options (a list of arcs in no particular order), and two messages:

1. Activate-A-Random-Arc: When this message is received, the state generates a random number between 1 and the number of arcs in Arc-Options. Then it returns the arc which has that Index number.

2. Activate-And-Return-Next-State: Receipt of this message results in the following actions:

   a. The Option-State sends itself the message Activate-A-Random-Arc, which returns a particular member of Arc-Options.
   b. It then sends to the returned arc (also encoded as an object) the message Activate-And-Rtrn-Destination-State. This returns a state, which will be the next state to visit after the current Option-State. It is the activation of the arc in this second step that generates text for the printer, if any.

In an object-oriented language, the programmer has the ability to create instances of a particular object type, and thereby populate his program with a set of such instances. Each instance has the slot names and messages *generic* to the object type, and slot values which are *unique* to that instance.

7.4. Overview of the Implementation

As mentioned above, in the transition net model, states are connected by arcs. Traversal through an ATN entails moving from state to state, across arcs. The objects required for TEXTNET are:

- states
  - Start-State
  - Pop-State
  - Cond-State
  - Option-State
  - Sequence-State
- arcs
  - Text-Arc
  - Function-Arc
  - Jump-Arc
  - Push-Arc
  - Endsequence-Arc

TEXTNET is built from these objects, plus one further object: Prose-Fact. Each net is designed to express (in prose form) some information which the system-builder wants to communicate to the user. As will be explained in detail below, the Prose-Fact object allows the system builder to pass this information to the net in a packaged form, rather than making such information global to the entire system.

Each net has one Start-State, and one Pop-State. Traversal of a network begins on the Start-State and ends when the Pop-State is reached. Separate networks can be arranged hierarchically by using Push-Arcs. When a Push-Arc is traversed the system "pushes" down to a "lower" network, which can be seen as a text generation subroutine. When that network has been traversed the system "pops" back up to continue in the original network.

7.5. Operational Description of the Objects

7.5.1. Prose Fact

Overview

The Prose-Fact object is used to pass information to nets. This object allows the system builder to reduce the number of global variables in a system with a large number of nets. The initialization message to any net includes a list called "prose-facts", which is a list of Prose-Fact instances. In this way, the facts required by a net can be passed to it at time of its activation. The Prose-Fact object has two slots (no messages).

Slots

1. Key: A primitive data type of the programming language, e.g., a string or a LISP atom.
2. Value: Some information stored with the key.

Consequently, the prose-facts which are passed in to a net are of the form ((key1 *value1*) (key2 *value2*) ... (keyN *valueN*)). The number of Prose-Facts passed to a net is arbitrary. At one extreme, every concept to be discussed might be packaged into a separate prose-fact before the information is passed to the net. At the other extreme, this separation of concepts might be "postponed" by using a single prose-fact containing a complex data structure. The net's Start-State must then separate the concepts before discussing them.

7.5.2. Start-State

Overview

A Start-State is the most complex of the TEXTNET states because it has several responsibilities: (1) it receives and identifies the 'facts' which this net needs to express, (2) it creates a set of local variables which can be used by states and arcs in the net during traversal, and finally (3) it coordinates traversal of the net. Because of these responsibilities, the slots and messages of a Start-State are complex, and require more explanation than other states.

Slots

1. Initialization-Fn: This slot contains the name of a function. This function is not a message. (That would make it generic to all Start-States.) This function is unique to each net (since there is a unique Start-State for each net). Each net needs to be able to express its own set of facts, in its own way. The Initialization-Fn provides a way of doing two things: 1) Unpacking the prose-facts, and identifying the facts which this net needs to know. 2) Setting up variables local to this net, which can be accessed and used by this net in its operation. This function is written by

the system builder (at the time that nets are being built for an application) to do the following:

a. Take one argument: "prose-facts". This is a list, each item of which is an instance of the object Prose-Fact. (Each net expects to find certain 'keys' among the prose-facts that are sent to it in the initial Genprose message. Genprose is discussed below under messages.)
b. Inspect the "prose-facts", identifying those keys that it anticipates finding.
c. Set up local variables that will be accessed and used by this net.
d. Send itself (i.e., this Start-State) the message Hop-Until-Pop.

The overall effect of evaluating this function is to initialize variables which will be needed by the net during its operation. The system builder can create any variables desired, simply by making them local variables within the Start-State's Initialization-Fn. Since the message Hop-Until-Pop (described below under messages) is sent within the body of the Initialization-Fn, these variables are also in effect for the duration of the Hop-Until-Pop function. Hop-Until-Pop coordinates the traversal of the net. When encountering a Pop-State, it finishes execution, returning control to the Initialization-Fn, which then relinquishes control as well, terminating the activity of this net.

2. State-Following-Start: A pointer to whatever state immediately follows the Start-State.

3. The-State-To-Activate-Next: This slot is used by the system to keep track of where it is in net traversal. It always contains a pointer to some state; the pointer changes as the net is traversed.

Messages

1. Genprose: This message takes one argument, "prose-facts", which is a list of Prose-Fact objects. This message does the following:

   a. Set The-State-To-Activate-Next equal to State-Following-Start.
   b. Call Initialization-Fn, with prose-facts as the argument.

2. Hop-Until-Pop: This message takes one argument: prose-facts, a list of Prose-Fact instances. This function should do the following:

```
While The-State-To-Activate-Next is NOT a Pop-State do
   Send the message: Activate-And-Return-Next-State
      to the slot The-State-To-Activate-Next,
      and
   Reset The-State-To-Activate-Next to whatever is returned.
```

7.5.3. Pop-State

Overview

This object is as very simple: it has no slots, and no messages. In each net, there must be one Start-State, an arbitrary number of intermediate states, and one Pop-State. The Hop-Until-Pop message (described above) continually looks for the Pop-State, and terminates as soon as one is identified. (In most object-oriented languages it is straightforward to determine whether an object is of a particular type, or class.)

7.5.4. Cond-State

Overview

This state typically examines one or more of the variables local to the net (recall that these variables are initialized by the Initialization-Fn of the Start-State) and conditionally chooses to traverse one of its arcs, depending upon what variable values it finds. A simple use of a Cond-State would be to assess whether a plural description is needed. For example, state B in Fig. 7-1 is a Cond-State. The message Return-Next-Arc-Index (described below under messages) might check a local variable, and if it contains a single item then return the "is" arc. (If the system builder wants to specify a single arc to be traversed, without any choice, then there should be only a single arc in the Conditional-Arcs slot, and the Return-Next-Arc-Index slot contains simply the integer 1, corresponding to the index on that arc.)

Slots

1. Conditional-Arcs: This slot contains a list of arcs which are defined by the net builder as he creates the net. Only one of these arcs will be used each time the Cond-State is activated. The choice of which arc to traverse is made by a procedure stored in the slot Return-Next-Arc-Index, as described below.

2. Return-Next-Arc-Index: This slot contains a function, which takes no arguments, and returns an integer between 1 and the number of Conditional-Arcs. (A safety check should assure that only values within those bounds can be returned by this function.) This is a second situation in which the system builder writes a function in the process of building nets for an application (the first situation, mentioned above, was for the Initialization-Fn slot in the Start-State).

Message

1. Activate-And-Return-Next-State: Receipt of this message results in these actions:

    a. Evaluate Return-Next-Arc-Index, which returns an index (integer).
    b. Identify the member of Conditional-Arcs which has that Index, (generating an error message if it is out of bounds).
    c. Send that arc the message Activate-And-Rtrn-Destination-State, (this message is known to all arcs in the TEXTNET scheme) returning some state in the net, which then becomes the return value for this function as well.

7.5.5. Option-State

Overview

When this state is activated, it chooses one of its arcs to traverse by random selection. It then activates that arc.

Slot

1. Arc-Options: This is a list of arcs, in no particular order.

Messages

1. Activate-A-Random-Arc: When this message is received, the state generates a random number between 1 and the number of arcs in Arc-Options. Then it returns the arc which has that Index number. (In many circumstances, it will prove useful to prevent the state from using the same arc consecutively in order to assure diversity in adjacent portions of the text output.)

2. Activate-And-Return-Next-State: Receipt of this message results in the following actions:

    a. Send itself (the Option-State) the message Activate-A-Random-Arc, which returns a particular member of Arc-Options.
    b. Send that particular arc the message Activate-And-Rtrn-Destination-State. This returns a state, which will be the next state visited after the current Option-State.

7.5.6. Sequence-State

Overview

A Sequence-State provides the facility to express a sequence of items, joined by natural phrasing. A typical set of Sequence-Arcs might contain text arcs "first," "second," "third," "in addition," and "also,". When a Sequence-State is activated, it chooses (in sequential order) one of its Sequence-Arcs to traverse. The state must therefore keep track, between activations, of the arc it traversed last. The system builder can store any number of Sequence-Arcs in the Sequence-State, but there is always the chance that the sequence of items to be described will be greater than the number of Sequence-Arcs provided. As a result, by convention this state iterates through its Sequence-Arcs and then continues to use the last arc for every activation until it receives the message End-Of-Sequence-Announcement (described below under messages). At that time, it re-initializes to the first arc again and is ready to start anew.

Slots

1. Sequence-Arcs: A list of arcs. As described below, all arcs in TEXTNET have an Index slot. Sequence-Arcs are assigned Index numbers which indicate the order in which they are to be used.

2. Endsequence-Jump-Arc: A Jump-Arc which is traversed when the state receives the message End-Of-Sequence-Announcement.

3. Index-Of-Next-Arc-To-Activate: This slot contains an integer, a counter with value between 1 and the number of arcs in the Sequence-Arcs slot.

4. Sequence-Just-Ended: This slot contains a boolean value, either True or False.

Messages

1. Initialize: When this message is received, the Index-Of-Next-Arc-To-Activate slot is set to 1, and the Sequence-Just-Ended slot is set to False.

2. End-Of-Sequence-Announcement: When this message is received, the Sequence-Just-Ended slot is set to True.

3. Fetch-The-Next-Seq-Arc-To-Activate: When this message is received, the following is done:

IF Sequence-Just-Ended = True, THEN do

a. Send itself the message Initialize.
b. Return the Endsequence-Jump-Arc.

ELSE IF Sequence-Just-Ended = False THEN do

a. If this state has never been initialized, then do so.
b. If the value of Index-Of-Next-Arc-To-Activate is less than the number of arcs in Sequence-Arcs, then increment that value by 1. (Otherwise leave the counter as is.)
c. Return that arc which has Index equal to Index-Of-Next-Arc-To-Activate.

4. Activate-And-Return-Next-State: Receipt of this message results in the following actions:

   a. Send itself the message Fetch-The-Next-Seq-Arc-To-Activate, returning an arc.
   b. Send that arc the message Activate-And-Rtrn-Destination-State. (This returns a state, which becomes the return value for this message as well.)

Operational descriptions of the *state* objects has been given above. The various types of *arc* objects are now described.

7.5.7. Push-Arc

Overview

A Push-Arc allows the creation of a hierarchy of nets. When a Push-Arc is traversed, the system "pushes" down to a lower net, and temporarily suspends processing of the upper net. When the Pop-State of the lower net is encountered, the system "pops" back up and continues. This allows a higher net to frame the discussion and pass control to a lower net for specific discussion of individual components of the larger discussion. For example, the lower nets might each be paragraphs within a larger prose discussion.

Slots

1. Destination: This is a pointer to the next state which is to be reached after this Push-Arc is traversed. (The lower net will generate prose

between the state of origin and the Destination.)

2. Index: All arcs have an Index identifier which is used as described above in the discussion of states.

3. Pushto-Name: This is the *global* name of the lower network's Start-State. The only global names in TEXTNET are the names of the Start-States of individual nets.

4. Fncall-That-Builds-N-Rtrns-Facts: This slot contains the name of a function which builds a list of "prose-facts". This list contains the information which the lower net will need in order to express the ideas that it is intended to express. There can be any number of Prose-Fact within "prose-facts". A Push-Arc sends the message Genprose to the lower net's Start-State, with prose-facts as the argument to that message.

Message

1. Activate-And-Rtrn-Destination-State: Receipt of this message causes the following actions:

   a. The function contained in the slot Fncall-That-Builds-N-Rtrns-Facts is evaluated.
   b. The message Genprose is sent to the Start-State of the lower net. This Start-State can be found by the system because the Pushto-Name is a global, which points to that Start-State. The argument of the message is the list "prose-facts" which was returned by action (a).

7.5.8. Jump-Arc

Overview

Activation of a Jump-Arc results in immediate traversal to the Destination state, without side effects. These arcs are used to bypass text which need not be output in certain situations. It is a way of "jumping" around an intermediate set of states and arcs.

Slots

1. Index: An integer.
2. Destination: Pointer to the next state in the net.

Message

1. Activate-And-Rtrn-Destination-State: Upon receipt of this message, the value of the Destination slot is immediately returned.

7.5.9. Text-Arc

Overview

When this arc is traversed, a text string is generated. This is one of the most widely used type of arcs.

Slots

1. Text: This slot contains a text string.
2. Index: An integer.
3. Destination: Pointer to the next state in the net.

Message

1. Activate-And-Rtrn-Destination-State: When a Text-Arc receives this message it does two things:
   a. The text string is sent to the printing buffer.
   b. The Destination state is returned.

7.5.10. Endsequence-Arc

Overview

The Endsequence-Arc has a very specific purpose. It's sole use is to signal a Sequence-State to reinitialize itself when there are no more items in the sequence it is currently processing. A deliberate termination of the sequence is needed if that sequence-arc is ever to be reused (to generate another sequence of arcs.)

Slots

1. Index: An integer.
2. Destination: Pointer to the next state in the net, which in this case *must* be a sequence state.

Message

1. Activate-And-Rtrn-Destination-State: Receipt of this message results in two actions:

a. The Destination state is sent the message End-Of-Sequence-Announcement.
b. The Destination state is returned.

7.5.11. Function-Arc

Overview

Traversal of a Function-Arc causes evaluation of a pre-defined function. Arcs of this type allow the system builder to generate material for prose from more complex function calls than simply pre-defined text strings. For example, this function could use local variables for computation.

Slots

1. Fncall-That-Rtrns-1-Lispitem-For-Printing: A pre-defined function, which does just that: it returns one Lispitem to be sent to the printer buffer.
2. Index: An integer.
3. Destination: Pointer to the next state in the net.

Message

1. Activate-And-Rtrn-Destination-State: Receipt of this message should cause three actions:

   a. The procedure contained in the slot Fncall-That-Rtrns-1-Lispitem-For-Printing is evaluated.
   b. That lispitem is sent to the printer buffer.
   c. The Destination state is returned.

7.6. Discussion

How does the TEXTNET approach[8] compare to other well-known projects in generating text such as the EMYCIN translator [Buchanan 84] or natural language

[8] As described in [Miller 86], the PROSENET approach was later augmented by the use of so-called "expressive frames" to allow more flexibility in structuring the prose output at the paragraph level then is currently afforded solely by TEXTNET. In the Roundsman system, TEXTNET offers considerable power and flexibility. Once a system designer has implemented TEXTNET and become comfortable with it, he could readily then add the expressive frame capability if he desired.

research such as that of Weiner [Weiner 80] and McKeown [McKeown 85]?

The EMYCIN approach is to translate code directly to text. Procedures and their arguments are translated into text strings which consequently reflect the procedural logic of the code. TEXTNET nets are not designed to translate code directly. TEXTNET is concerned with a certain set of conclusions drawn by the expert system and not with the procedural code itself. First the system draws inferences, and only then does it pass conclusions to TEXTNET in order to produce text. If the system-builder feels that something should to be explained by TEXTNET, then the system must save that item as a conclusion.

An advantage of the EMYCIN translator approach is that if the program code is altered, the text explanation will *automatically* be modified appropriately. Of course, it may not be necessary to change the TEXTNET network either: the nets will need alteration if the form of the conclusions changes, but this may not always be true simply because procedural code has changed. Nevertheless, it is true that the TEXTNET nets anticipate a certain form of conclusions. If that form should change as the program evolves, the nets must be altered accordingly. It is usually straightforward to build new nets or alter old ones.

It is difficult for a direct-translation approach like EMYCIN to capture the subtleties of language. Introductory phrasing, bridging comments, and variations of wording are powerful aspects of good exposition. Theoretically, there is no reason these could not be achieved with direct translation. Nevertheless, in practice these features are difficult to achieve because the design does not make it easy to see the overall picture. TEXTNET's Push-Arcs allow the designer to consider the text structure at various levels of detail, and to refine the prose one level at a time. Sequence-States and Option-States make it easy to achieve introductory phrasing and variations of wording. Also, arcs and states can be pulled apart and re-assembled easily. This facilitates the rapid development of the prose effect desired by the system builder.

Weiner's research focusses on generating explanations that do not appear overly complex to the user [Weiner 80]. His system, named BLAH, contains a knowledge base of assertions and justifications. BLAH can be queried (a) to choose between two assertions, (b) whether some assertion is believed, or (c) why an assertion is believed. To respond, the system first constructs a "reasoning tree" consisting of statements and reasons which branch out to "leaf" node assertions from the knowledge base. The system then "prunes" the tree to eliminate what the user knows, breaks up the tree if it considered too large for a single response, and finally generates text from the remaining trees and subtrees.

McKeown's research in natural language generation is a much more ambitious research project that TEXTNET. Her system (TEXT) is a natural language interface to a database system which responds to questions about the structure of the database with answers about a paragraph in length. McKeown's main research goals were to delineate a formal model of discourse strategies rather than to develop a practical text generation system. Accordingly, less effort has gone into optimizing the implementation. In any case, the program design is more complex than many expert system builders will want for a text generation module.

Research into natural language text generation (such as McKeown's and Weiner's) may progress to the point where a sophisticated model of discourse can be used as a practical component of an expert system. In the interim, a more straightforward approach like TEXTNET may nevertheless allow an expert system considerable flexibility and power in its prose expression.

Chapter 8

Extended Examples and Evaluation

The first eight sections of this chapter provide examples of Roundsman in action: each section includes one example critique followed by a discussion. Section 8.9 presents the results of an evaluation of Roundsman's performance, and a discussion of those results.

In each example Roundsman is critiquing a proposal for the surgical management of a particular patient's breast cancer. Since the critiques are rich in clinical detail, it must be re-emphasized that Roundsman is currently a research project. These critiques are an important first step toward providing a new type of computer-based decision support, but they can *not* be used as advice for actual clinical decisions at this time. Indeed, the trained clinician may notice comments which are clinically controversial or possibly incorrect. Further research and development are needed, as well as more intensive collaboration with the medical experts in the domain.

Each example consists of (a) a statement of the clinical context (a description of the patient and the physician's treatment proposal) (b) a verbatim transcript of Roundsman's critique of one particular study in light of that clinical context and (c) a discussion of certain aspects of the example critique. For each clinical context Roundsman usually selected between three and five studies for discussion. The output in these examples is typical of Roundsman's performance and the only "selection" involved was making sure that the examples included biomedical reports from a range of experimental designs, from several time periods, and that the examples show how a study's critique changes for different clinical contexts. The discussion of example 1 is more detailed in order to set the stage for the later examples.

8.1. Example 1

Clinical Context:

- *For a woman whose* tumor size is T1a, axillary lymph nodes are N1a, is premenopausal, age 45, unknown axillary node histology (this cannot be known until after the surgery) and no metastases.
- *Treatment proposal of* surgical wide excision (& axillary dissection) plus adjuvant radiotherapy plus adjuvant chemotherapy if axillary node histology is subsequently positive.

Roundsman's Critique:

Fisher85a was a randomized, controlled trial conducted at multiple NSABP centers. Subjects were assigned to verified wide excision with axillary dissection and adjuvant radiotherapy (N= 373) or the alternative therapy of verified wide excision with axillary dissection (N= 358). For patients who underwent the first protocol the proportion free of ipsilateral breast recurrence at five years was equal to 0.9, overall survival at five years turned out to be 0.91 and recurrence-free survival at five years was 0.81. Under the second protocol the proportion free of ipsilateral breast recurrence at five years turned out to be 0.77, overall survival at five years was 0.9 and recurrence-free survival at five years was equal to 0.68.

Are these results relevant to your patient? It is encouraging that first, the adjuvant modality you propose was specified for this study as well (chemotherapy given if axillary nodes are path. positive). Second, this study population is quite similar to your patient (the women in this group had T sizes ranging up to T2a but excision margins were verified free of tumor). We suspect it makes little difference that the intervention was somewhat nonstandard (they did not radiate supraclavicular nodes). More troublesome is that the study population was probably in a better prognostic stratum than your patient (this study stratum was defined by negative axillary node histology; about 40% of clinical stage I patients like yours will have positive histology).

What is the validity of the data? It helps that first, the investigator is reliable (the NSABP trials are first-rate, e.g., participating physicians must be certified by Fisher). Second, controls were randomly assigned. The results are weakened because one of their outcomes was a bit nonstandard (recurrence in the ipsilateral breast was NOT counted as a local recurrence).

More than one outcome type is reported, but strictly on the basis of five-year results in recurrence-free survival, your suggested therapy seems best (although not all results agree). The close fit of your patient, considered together with the the excellent methodology probably would not alter that statistical conclusion. The first protocol mentioned (which is close to your proposed plan) appears to be the better one.

This example illustrates several reasons why the clinical literature is an interesting problem area for employing computer-based decision support:

- Complexity of experimental design: This trial (NSABP protocol 6) compares three different interventions in parallel: (1) total mastectomy, (2) excision ("lumpectomy") and (3) excision plus radiation. In certain subsets of each group, chemotherapy was used. Several endpoints were reported: overall survival, recurrence-free survival and ipsilateral breast recurrence. For the physician requesting this consultation, Roundsman has decided to highlight a comparison of intervention arms 2 and 3.

Proper analysis of the results is complicated by the fact that the patients used to compute the results of intervention 2 are not the same when interventions 1 and 2 are compared as when when interventions 3 and 2 are compared (as is discussed more fully in example 2). This design complexity has a domain-specific motivation which is of more interest to oncologists than computer scientists. The important point is that even in just presenting the first paragraph, Roundsman has already done a significant amount of work for the physician by sifting through the numerous interventions, subsets of patients and endpoints in order to present *selective* portions of a complex body of experimental evidence. Next comes Roundsman's principal focus: the further subjective assessment of the relevance of *those selective portions* to the physician's clinical case.

- Clinical details of the study: Although certain clinical details are all crucial to an intelligent assessment of the study for clinical purposes, it is practically impossible for a physician to recall these details months or years after reading the article. The cost of refreshing these details is a line-by-line reading of a lengthy technical article. For example, certain clinical conditions had to exist before chemotherapy was given (paragraph 2), several T (tumor) sizes were allowed in this group of women studied, but excision margins were verified free of tumor (paragraph 2), supraclavicular nodes (i.e, lymph nodes located above the collar-bone) were not exposed to radiation (paragraph 2), and the definition of "local recurrence" excluded recurrences in the breast which had the original tumor (paragraph 3). Thus Roundsman brings to light certain clinical details which may help the physician use this experimental evidence for his purposes.

- Relevance of clinical detail to the physician making a particular management decision: The second and third paragraphs not only offer subjective judgments about which clinical details of the study should be explicitly juxtaposed against the physician's patient and treatment decision, but in addition offer subjective judgments about the *importance* of any mismatch when using the study to discuss the management problem under consideration. For example, the fact that the physician *also* plans to use chemotherapy if the axillary node histology turns out to be positive (paragraph 2) makes it easier to say that this report can provide some support for this management decision. Irradiation of supraclavicular nodes is judged to be a minor detail whatever the physician chooses to do.

8.2. Example 2

Example 2 shows how Roundsman's critique of Fisher85a (the study discussed in example 1) changes when the physician's patient is different.

Clinical Context:

- *For a woman with* tumor size T1a, axillary lymph node status N1b, pre-menopausal, age 45 unknown axillary node histology and no metastases.
- *Treatment proposal of* surgical wide excision (& axillary dissection) plus adjuvant radiotherapy plus adjuvant chemotherapy if axillary node histology is subsequently positive.

Roundsman's Critique:

Fisher85a was a randomized, controlled trial performed by investigators at multiple NSABP centers. Patients were randomized to wide excision (& axillary dissection) and adjuvant radiotherapy and adjuvant chemotherapy (N= 229) or another protocol which was total mastectomy (& axillary dissection) and adjuvant chemotherapy (N= 224). For patients who underwent the first protocol the overall survival at five years turned out to be 0.75 and recurrence-free survival at five years was equal to 0.58. Under the second protocol the overall survival at five years was 0.66 and recurrence-free survival at five years was equal to 0.58.

How do these data apply to your patient? We are not particularly concerned that the intervention was somewhat nonstandard (they did not radiate supraclavicular nodes). More troublesome is that first, there were modifications to one intervention (in the excision arm, women with positive margins received total mastectomy, but remained in the 'excision' group). Second, the study population was in a worse prognostic stratum compared to your patient (this study stratum was defined by positive axillary node histology; about 40% of clinical stage II patients like yours will have negative histology).

How much confidence can we have in the experimental results? It's good to see that first, the investigator is reliable (the NSABP trials are first-rate, e.g., participating physicians must be certified by Fisher). Second, controls were randomly assigned. The results are weakened because one of their outcomes was a bit nonstandard (recurrence in the ipsilateral breast was NOT counted as a local recurrence).

Looking selectively at five-year results in recurrence-free survival, those two interventions look equivalent (the other results generally agree). The 'relevance' problems detailed above, considered together with the excellent methodology probably would not alter that statistical conclusion. Consequently, a choice between these two approaches might be made on the basis of morbidity (cosmesis, etc.) rather than cure.

In example 2, Roundsman's critique has changed in several ways from that shown in example 1:

- Dealing with the complexity of experimental design: The patient in example 2 has worse disease than the woman considered in example 1. This patient has stage II breast cancer, and it is more controversial whether excision is a safe surgical approach for her disease than for the woman in example 1. Consequently, in example 2 Roundsman chooses to focus its discussion on a comparison of a different *surgical* approach, rather than a comparison of the omission or addition of radiation (as in example 1). As mentioned earlier, Fisher85a studied three different interventions in parallel, so for this example Roundsman has presented evidence concerning total mastectomy versus wide excision.

- Relevance of clinical detail to the physician making a particular management decision: As mentioned in the discussion of example 1, the patients used to determine the results of intervention 2 are not the same when interventions 1 and 2 are compared as when interventions 3 and 2 are compared. Understanding this point requires attention to clinical detail: the Fisher85a protocol specified that women entered into the excision arm *must* have the margins of their excision verified free of tumor. If margins are *not* free, then the woman went on to have a total mastectomy. For the analysis of the excision group versus the total mastectomy group, women who failed to have clear margins (and thus received total mastectomies) *were counted as members of the excision group.* Why? To exclude them would have biased the results: the total mastectomy group did not check excision margins; excluding unclear margins from the excision group would exclude women with bigger tumors, making the results look better than they should. This clinical detail is brought to the attention of the physician in sentence 3 of paragraph 2 in the critique just above.

  One might then ask why this clinical detail was not mentioned in the critique in example 1? This was not done because in comparing "excision" versus "excision plus radiotherapy" (discussed in example 1), women who fail to have clean margins and therefore receive total mastectomy *are* excluded from the count. The critique in example 1 need not concern the physician with clinical detail(s) of the study which do not impact upon the clinical context he currently is considering.

8.3. Example 3

Example 3 shows what a consultation with Roundsman would look like if the date were 1967. In order to do this Roundsman is restricted to publications which appeared prior to 1968. Also, the date of the consultation (a system variable) is set to "1967". In 1967, total mastectomy was being advocated by some physicians but it was a controversial management decision: the consensus was that doing less than a radical mastectomy endangered the life of a woman with breast cancer. In the example session (below) the physician is planning to use total mastectomy and one of the studies Roundsman discusses is Kaee65, which reports on a comparison of total mastectomy versus a form of radical mastectomy.

Clinical Context: year= 1967

- *For a woman with* tumor status T1a, clinical node status N1b, pre-menopausal, age 45, and no indication of metastases.
- *Treatment proposal of* total mastectomy with axillary dissection.

Roundsman's Critique:

Kaee65 was a randomized, controlled trial carried out at Copenhagen. Subjects were assigned to total mastectomy and adjuvant radiotherapy (N= 70) or to treatment with extended radical mastectomy (N= 65). For patients who underwent the first protocol the recurrence-free survival at five years was 0.36 and overall survival at five years turned out to be 0.46. Under the second protocol the recurrence-free survival at five years was 0.37 and overall survival at five years turned out to be 0.46.

How do these data apply to your patient? It is encouraging that this study population is quite similar to your patient (it was a clinical stage II population). It's probably not too important that their therapy was suboptimal (orthovoltage 4500 rads over 4 wks is a bit low), or that the intervention was somewhat nonstandard (the 'radical' mastectomy was somewhat more extensive than Halstedian radical but for this analysis it stands for the 'radical mastectomy' group). More troublesome is that first, the study protocol included a modality beyond your proposed treatment (unless you use adjuvant radiotherapy as they did in this study, it is questionable whether these results can be used for your case). Second, these patients are from a broader prognostic group than one would like (group definition, 'operable minus stage I', captured primarily stage II's but also some III's since T size was not a criterion).

What is the validity of the data? It helps that controls were randomly assigned (using an odd number/even number scheme). The results are weakened because first, uncontrolled treatment variables might skew the results (total mastectomies were performed at one hospital and radicals at another: how comparable was post-operative nursing etc?). Second, a selection bias might have been introduced (criteria for 'operability' determined by biopsy in the radical mx. patients but by physical exam for total mx. patients). Third, a large number of eligible patients were subsequently excluded (about 20% of the eligible patients in each arm were excluded -- starts to jeopardize group comparability).

When the evidence is isolated to five-year results in recurrence-free survival, those two interventions look equivalent (the other results generally agree). The mismatch of your particular clinical situation, considered together with the methodological weaknesses mentioned earlier however, leads us to think that the results are indecisive for your purposes. Adhering to the standard of care (radical mastectomy) would probably be most appropriate.

Example 3 demonstrates how Roundsman's critique might help the physician faced with the clinical problem described above. First, Roundsman identifies Kaee65 as one body of potential experimental evidence regarding the less conventional approach (total mastectomy) for this patient. Second, Roundsman generates a discussion of this publication which might otherwise be possible only by critically reading of the paper *with this particular patient and treatment proposal in mind.*

- Complexity of experimental design: As in the previous examples, Roundsman presents the sample sizes, endpoints measured, and the outcome proportions observed selectively: the critique discusses only that patient group whose characteristics are closest to the patient.

- Clinical details of the study: In paragraph 2 we learn that the investigators used orthovoltage radiation, that the radical mastectomy was a more "extended" surgical procedure than usual, and that the group definition for these patients admitted some women with stage III breast disease. Paragraph 3 informs us that after randomization the two groups of women were treated at totally different hospitals and that a sizeable number of patients were later excluded from the analysis. It is important to realize that these details are *not* a mere reiteration of the "methods" section of this publication. There are many technical details discussed in any such paper. Roundsman discusses only those clinical details which the collaborating oncologist feels are significant for a critical appraisal of the study (and are therefore included in Roundsman's internal representation for Kaee65).

- Relevance of clinical detail to the management problem being considered: Roundsman provides a rough *calibration* of the seriousness of various mismatches between the study details and the clinical problem facing the physician. For example, the fact that the radical mastectomy was "extended" (paragraph 2) is not thought to threaten the applicability of this study to the physician's case, whereas the absence of radiotherapy in the physician's plan is judged to be a "more troublesome" problem (paragraph 2). These are *subjective* assessments which are based upon the clinical judgment of a collaborating oncologist. It is a deliberate design decision that Roundsman makes the clinical context of these subjective judgments clear to the user of the program: the physician-user must be able to understand the underlying issues and override the machine if he disagrees about any of the subjective judgments.

It is interesting that failure to add radiotherapy to mastectomy, cited in the critique of example 3 as a serious omission, is in later years [Fisher 80] judged to make no difference to patient survival. The injection of this new scientific knowledge (via clinical studies) highlights two advantages of Roundsman's approach: (a) The prose critique of Kaee65 includes enough clinical detail to recognize if a judgment has become obsolete. (b) Roundsman generates its critiques dynamically, on the basis of flexible data structures. These data structures can be altered to reflect the changing state of knowledge: to update Roundsman after publication of [Fisher 80] requires only that one of Roundsman's *distance-estimator* objects be given new slot values for "dp-change" and "specifics". If instead, the critiques of Kaee65 and of *all studies which examined the combination of radiotherapy with total mastectomy* were "canned text", then *each* such canned critique would require rewriting when the obsolescence was encountered.

8.4. Example 4

Example 4 shows how Roundsman's critique of Kaee65 changes when the physicia is dealing with a *different clinical problem* from example 3. (The consultation yea is still 1967.) In example 4, the physician proposes using adjuvant radiotherapy i addition to the mastectomy proposed in example 3. Furthermore, the patient's brea disease in example 4 is less advanced than the breast disease of the patient discusse in example 3.

Clinical Context: year = 1967

- *For a woman with* tumor status T1a, clinical node status N1a (axillary lymph nodes palpable but thought not to contain tumor), pre-menopausal, age 45, and no indications of metastases.
- *Treatment proposal of* total mastectomy with axillary dissection plus adjuvant radiotherapy.

Roundsman's Critique:

> Kaee65 was a randomized, controlled trial conducted at Copenhagen. Patients were randomized to total mastectomy and adjuvant radiotherapy (N= 149) or the alternative therapy of extended radical mastectomy (N= 141). In the group which received the first protocol the recurrence-free survival at five years was equal to 0.67 and overall survival at five years turned out to be 0.67. Under the second protocol the recurrence-free survival at five years was 0.68 and overall survival at five years was equal to 0.68.
>
> How well does the study generalize to your particular patient? It is encouraging that your patient fits the study population extremely well (the group studied was clinical stage I). We are not particularly concerned that their therapy was suboptimal (orthovoltage 4500 rads over 4 wks is a bit low), or that the intervention was somewhat nonstandard (the 'radical' mastectomy was somewhat more extensive than Halstedian radical but for this analysis it stands for the 'radical mastectomy' group).
>
> [*The third paragraph of example 4 is basically the same as that of example 3, and is omitted from this transcript.*]
>
> Looking selectively at five-year results in recurrence-free survival, those two interventions look equivalent (the other results generally agree). The close fit of your patient, considered together with the reasonably good methodology probably would not alter that statistical conclusion. Consequently, a choice between these two approaches might be made on the basis of morbidity (cosmesis, etc.) rather than cure.

In example 4 Roundsman's critique differs in several from that of example 3:

- Complexity of experimental design: Since the patient in example 4 differs from the patient of example 3, Roundsman discusses a different stratum. This is reflected in the larger sample sizes (more stage I patients were recruited than stage II patients) and the changed outcome proportions in the first paragraph. (Compare example 4 to example 3.)

- Relevance of clinical detail to the management problem being considered: Unlike the critique of example 3, this critique does not warn that the absence of adjuvant radiotherapy in the physician's plan makes it difficult to use the results of Kaee65 (since the physician's plan includes radiotherapy). Also, Roundsman's selection of a different patient group results in a change in the second sentence of paragraph 2 and allows Roundsman to omit any complaint about the overly broad prognostic group (as in paragraph 2 of example 3). These changes -- which stem from considering the study in light of a *different patient* and a *different treatment combination* -- in turn impact upon the conclusions of the last paragraph.

8.5. Example 5

Clinical studies are not all randomized controlled trials. Indeed, when a management issue is highly controversial, much of the evidence is often in the form of *case series* reports. That is, patients are treated in a single manner, and their outcome is then informally compared (either implicitly or explicitly) to the usual outcome expected with other treatments. Despite their methodological weaknesses as experiments, case series reports continue to play an important role in the clinical literature (see, for example, two other case series reports [Levene 77, Hellman 80] which are represented in Roundsman's library). In example 5, Roundsman discusses Haagensen69, a large case series report. Dr. Haagensen's publications were, at that time, the most respected medical advice available on the management of breast cancer.

Clinical Context: year = 1970

- *For a woman with* clinical tumor status T1a, clinical node status N1a, pre-menopausal, age 45 and no known metastases.
- *Treatment proposal of* radical mastectomy.

Roundsman's Critique:

Haagensen69 reports on a case series (without internal controls) study conducted at Columbia-Presbyterian, New York. 344 subjects received radical mastectomy and adjuvant radiotherapy. Overall survival at ten years was 0.69 and overall survival at five years was equal to 0.85.

How well does the study generalize to your particular patient? It is encouraging that this study population is quite similar to your patient (in this judgment we recognize that although they were N0-N1a like your patient, they included not only T1 but T2 and T3 as well). We are not particularly concerned that the intervention was somewhat nonstandard (few breast surgeons adhere strictly to Haagensen's strenuous procedure which entails a 5 hour operation), or that the intervention was nonuniform ('some' of the patients received radiotherapy, and some did not).

What is the validity of the data? Among the strongpoints we note that the investigator is reliable (Haagensen has more experience with breast cancer management than any physician in this country - he is widely respected). The results are weakened because first, there were no internal controls (but given this design, Haagensen strengthened it by including ALL consecutive patients, and not losing a single patient to follow-up). Second, patients were accrued over a rather long period (patients were entered between 1935 and 1951).

The first paragraph of this critique makes clear that (a) there are no internal controls in Haagensen69, and (b) the sample size is extremely large (especially for that time period). The second paragraph illustrates how Roundsman's distance-estimators handle *dependent parameters.* For example, tumor size and nodal status are correlated: as tumor size increases, the probability of having positive axillary nodes (N1b) increases. If the patient has a worse axillary node status than the study group, and also has a larger T (tumor) status, it would be "double-counting" to comment independently on those two mismatches. Consequently, these two patient characteristics are best handled simultaneously by one distance-estimator. In this example, that distance-estimator's conclusion is passed to TEXTNET which then produces the second sentence of paragraph 2 (above). In this example, Roundsman cannot offer a useful fourth paragraph contrasting two alternatives because there are no internal controls for comparison. This is consistent with the conventional manner in which case series information is used: implicit comparisons with information external to the study is more or less left to the reader.

8.6. Example 6

In examples 1-4 Roundsman discussed randomized, controlled studies. In example 5 Roundsman discussed a study that had no internal controls. Example 6 shows Roundsman critiquing yet a third type of clinical study: one with *non-randomized* internal controls. The publication discussed in this example appeared in the literature when radical mastectomy was the standard of care and surgical excision was used by only a small minority of surgeons.

Clinical Context: year = 1967

- *For a woman whose* clinical exam reveals tumor size T1a, axillary nodes thought to contain tumor (N1b) is pre-menopausal, age 45, and has no metastases.
- *Treatment proposal of* wide excision, axillary dissection and adjuvant

radiotherapy.

Roundsman's Critique:

Peters67 employed non-randomized controls in a study conducted at Princess Margaret Hospital, Toronto. A set of patients who were treated by wedge resection and adjuvant radiotherapy (N= 94) is contrasted to a second therapy group: radical mastectomy and adjuvant radiotherapy (N= 247). In the group which received the first protocol the overall survival at five years was 0.76. For patients who underwent the second protocol the overall survival at five years turned out to be 0.72.

How well does the study generalize to your particular patient? We are not particularly concerned that one modality you propose may not be quite like what was done in the study ('wedge resection' here indicates excisional biopsy, quadrant resection, or any technique to excise the primary). More troublesome is that the study population was probably in a better prognostic stratum than your patient (the study used a pooled clinical stage I and II - so that's a slightly better prognostic group than your patient).

How much confidence can we have in the experimental results? The results are weakened because first, choice of treatment was decided non-randomly (nor were subjects and controls matched on prognostic parameters). Second, patients were accrued over a rather long period (this is a retrospective study of patients treated between 1935 and 1960). Third, this is a wide stratum (it would have been preferable to separate stages I and II).

Considering the reported observations and sample size (see introductory paragraph), those two interventions look equivalent. The small mismatch of your particular clinical situation, considered together with the the large methodological weaknesses however, leads us to think that the results are indecisive for your purposes. Adhering to the standard of care (radical mastectomy) would probably be most appropriate.

In retrospect, the nearly equivalent proportions reported in paragraph 1 (above) have been borne out by later studies which compared mastectomy to excision (e.g., Fisher85a in examples 1 and 2). In this consultation, however, Roundsman is unable to confidently conclude that Peters67 provides enough support for the physician to deviate from more standard surgical approach (see last sentence of the concluding paragraph). The reasons for this lack of support are explained by Roundsman: the nonuniform nature of the intervention (paragraph 2), the broad stratum of patients lumped together for analysis (paragraph 2), the non-random experimental design (paragraph 3) and and the long accrual period (paragraph 3).

8.7. Example 7

Example 7 discusses a clinical study which appears to conflict with the results of certain other studies. The other studies [Veronesi 81, Fisher 85a] suggest that wide excision combined with radiotherapy is a safe alternative to mastectomy, especially for stage I patients. Example 7 discusses a 1983 publication which seems to suggest otherwise.

Clinical Context: year = 1985

- *For a woman who* is clinically assessed as tumor status T1a, nodal status N1a, post-menopausal, age 60, without known metastases.
- *Treatment proposal of* wide excision (& axillary dissection) plus adjuvant radiotherapy.

Roundsman's Critique:

> Hayward83 was a randomized, controlled trial conducted at Guy's Hospital, England. Patients were randomized to wide excision and adjuvant radiotherapy (N= 121) or the alternative therapy of radical mastectomy and adjuvant radiotherapy (N= 132). In the group which received the first protocol the overall survival at five years turned out to be 0.72 and the proportion free of local or regional recurrence at five years was 0.75. Under the second protocol the overall survival at five years turned out to be 0.85 and the proportion free of local or regional recurrence at five years was equal to 0.93.
>
> How well does the study generalize to your particular patient? It is encouraging that your patient fits the study population extremely well (the group studied was clinical stage I). More troublesome is that their therapy was suboptimal (2500 rads of orthovoltage is suboptimal).
>
> What is the quality of the study? It helps that controls were randomly assigned.
>
> Considering the reported observations and sample size (see introductory paragraph), the other protocol appears superior to yours. The close fit of your patient suggests that you might be better off using an approach like the second protocol (described in the first paragraph) in lieu of the plan you proposed.

The fourth paragraph cautions the physician that, on the basis of this clinical trial, mastectomy appears to be superior to his plan of wide excision and radiation. Many clinicians feel that the low dose of radiation ruined this trial, and that if they had used higher doses it would have shown that wide excision plus radiation is a safe alternative to mastectomy. Nevertheless, there are today a number of physicians who view Hayward83, as well as a previous trial at Guy's Hospital [Atkins 72, Hayward 77], as good evidence that wide excision is unsafe. One prominent feature of medicine is "conflicting expertise": the honest disagreement among expert clinicians as to the correct course of action. It is only reasonable that underlying such conflicting expertise, there is conflicting *evidence* which can be interpreted in more than one way. A system like Roundsman should have explicit access to any such disagreement, and should be able to discuss the issues intelligibly.

8.8. Example 8

The last section of Chapter 3 previously described how a Roundsman critique is developed via the five steps shown in Fig. 1-1. The example critique used for the step-by-step exposition in Chapter 3 is a discussion of Veronesi81 for a physician who plans to use excision and radiotherapy for a woman with stage II breast cancer. Example 8 (below) illustrates how that critique (see page 44 of this book) changes when Roundsman discusses a different clinical problem:

Clinical Context:

- *For a woman whose* tumor status is T1a, clinical node status is N1a, is post-menopausal, age 65, without known metastases.
- *Treatment proposal of* wide excision plus radiotherapy and chemotherapy if axillary nodes are positive upon pathological examination.

Roundsman's Critique:

> Veronesi81 was a randomized, controlled trial carried out at the Cancer Institute in Milan. Patients were randomized to quadrantectomy and adjuvant radiotherapy and CMF for histology+ patients (N= 352) or another protocol which was radical mastectomy and CMF for histology+ patients (N= 349). Under the first protocol the overall survival at five years was equal to 0.9 and recurrence-free survival at five years was 0.84. In the group which received the second protocol the overall survival at five years was equal to 0.9 and recurrence-free survival at five years turned out to be 0.83.
>
> How do these data apply to your patient? It is encouraging that first, the adjuvant modality you propose was specified for this study as well (chemotherapy given if axillary nodes are path. positive). Second, your patient fits the study population extremely well (the group studied was clinical stage 1). We suspect it makes little difference that the intervention was somewhat nonstandard (quadrantectomy removes more

tissue than wide excision).

What is the validity of the data? It's good to see that controls were randomly assigned (and stratified by menopausal status before randomization).

More than one outcome type is reported, but strictly on the basis of five-year results in recurrence-free survival those two interventions look equivalent (the other results generally agree). The close fit of your patient suggests that a choice between your proposed therapy and the second protocol (see paragraph 1) might be made on the basis of morbidity (cosmesis, etc.) rather than cure.

Several aspects of this critique differ from the critique shown on page 44. The physician's plan to conditionally administer chemotherapy, and the clinical node status (N1a), are seen as reasons why in this case it *is* reasonable to use Veronesi81 as the basis for decision-making. In the example (in Chapter 3), Roundsman argued that the study could not be decisive evidence for the case at hand. As a result, the final paragraph of example 8 encourages the physician to use the results of Veronesi81 as support that his plan of wide excision will not endanger the life of his patient, and that decision-making criteria can therefore focus on other (non life-threatening) issues of morbidity such as the cosmetic cost, the trauma of surgery, and the local recurrence rate.

8.9. Evaluation

8.9.1. Introduction

This section discusses an evaluation of the Roundsman system. This was the first structured evaluation of Roundsman, so the number of cases is small and one of the two oncologist evaluators was the expert who assisted in the development of Roundsman. This study was intended to provide useful feedback and insights rather than formal statistical results.

Evaluating a decision support system may provide insight to the system builders but may also demonstrate to observers outside the project that the system attains certain performance standards. (See Chapter 8 of [Hayes-Roth 83] for a discussion of system evaluation.) If the system produces an "answer" for which there is a gold standard (e.g., an autopsy diagnosis) then a measure of correct performance is available. On the other hand, decision support systems may be of value not just because of an overall "answer", but for the capability to *explain* the basis for conclusions drawn, and for the degree to which the system's advice displays "common sense" about the problem domain [Teach 81]. For example, decision support systems for medical *management* must cope with the fact that there is frequently no gold-standard for the advice. Indeed, advice systems for medical management may be most useful precisely when reliable scientific knowledge about the effects of a new medication or a controversial procedure are not yet known, and consequently there is expert disagreement about the correct course of action. Evaluation of a medical advice system then, may focus on how well the system frames the problem and brings useful information (which may include conflicting data) to the attention of the user.

When asking clinicians to judge Roundsman's output, it is important to make clear the program's recognized limitations:

- Breadth of Roundsman's library:

    - Clinical: Roundsman currently represents studies only on the surgical and radiotherapeutic management of primary breast cancer. There is interesting experimental evidence which lies outside the scope of Roundsman's knowledge base (e.g., the literature evaluating the effects of various chemotherapeutic regimens; literature on the management of recurrent breast cancer).

    - Statistical: Roundsman does not currently include certain types of biomedical reports (e.g., cross-sectional studies).

- Depth of Roundsman's library: There may be pertinent reports which are not contained in the the Roundsman's system current library of 24 studies.

- Clinical heuristics: Roundsman is not designed to reason about subtle clinical issues such as tailoring therapy in the presence of a coexisting disease.

It was anticipated that problems with the program output might include the following:

- Phrasing and Style: Roundsman's ability to produce prose makes the performance of the system accessible to a broad clinical audience. Specifically, it allows oncologists to help us understand the strengths and weaknesses of the system. On the other hand, when an author re-reads a paper he has written earlier, he quite often feels that the phrasing could be improved, or that a somewhat different organization of the concepts would be better. Roundsman's prose will also encounter this kind of criticism.

- Content Incorrect: The evaluator may feel that a comment is flatly incorrect, or correct but inappropriate for the clinical context.

- Content Missing: The system may fail to make comments which, on the basis of its knowledge base and design goals, it should be capable of making.

8.9.2. Methods

Two oncologists, Robert Carlson and Frank Stockdale, graciously gave their time to evaluate the quality of Roundsman's output (a critique for a particular patient and treatment proposal).

The evaluation forms used by the oncologists are shown in Table 8-1 and Table 8-2. One copy of the form shown in Table 8-1 was used *each* time the evaluator wanted to make a change to some particular line of Roundsman's output. The form shown in Table 8-2 allowed the evaluator to make overall comments on the critique. The purpose of completing the evaluation forms is to identify *problems* with the critiques.

The goal of analyzing the evaluation forms is to identify the *problem source*. A listing of potential problem sources is shown in Table 8-4 (page 162).

The two evaluators chose material to review from a set of approximately 85 (previously-run) critiques. ("Critique" here means Roundsman's discussion of one study.) These 85 included nine different patient/plan scenarios and three different years: 1967, 1977 and 1985. (As described in section 6.1, Roundsman's knowledge base of publications was built chronologically and a consultation can be run on any year between 1948 and 1985. Example 3 in this chapter shows a consultation run with year set to 1967.) Evaluator A reviewed nine critiques (from among the 85) and evaluator B reviewed seven, for a total of sixteen separate reviews. They did not choose the same critiques to review.

8.9.3. Results

The number and type of corrections suggested by the reviewers is summarized in Table 8-3. Phrasing changes were deemed (by both oncologists) to be important issues in the quality of the critique. As is shown in Table 8-3, the oncologist who evaluated critiques J-P was more often concerned with phrasing and style errors than the oncologist who evaluated critiques A-I. The evaluators were similar in the

Use this page to suggest **Changes to a Particular Comment**

On Critique #_____, see comment marked #_____.

1. **Would suggest different phrasing**. (Circle as many as applicable.)
   a. Phrasing too vague: it is unclear what is being said.
   b. Does not use oncology terminology properly.
   c. Other (please specify):

Suggested phrasing:

2. **Disagree with the content of comment:**

```
Extent of disagreement:

                        1  2  3  4
                minor             severe
           correction             disagreement

Why you disagree:
```

3. Other:

Table 8-1: Form used for changes to a particular comment.

Use this page for an **Overall Assessment** of Critique #______

Problem with the style of the critique?

1. Material should be presented in a different order.

2. Paragraph(s) need a better topic sentence to orient the reader.

3. Other:

What's missing from the critique?

1. Additional population match issue:

2. Additional intervention match issue:

3. Additional comment(s) on the quality of the study:

4. Comment about interaction(s) between studies:

5. Other (please specify):

Table 8-2: Form used to note general problems of a critique.

	Size of Critique in Sentences	Phrasing Changes	Content Disagreements	Style Problems	Missing Comments
A	12	2	1	0	1
B	12	0	0	1	1
C	12	0	0	0	1
D	13	4	0	0	1
E	14	0	1	0	1
F	13	1	1	0	2
G	13	0	2	0	1
H	12	0	1	0	0
I	12	0	1	0	2
J	13	4	2	4	3
K	13	4	1	1	1
L	13	3	0	1	1
M	15	6	0	2	0
N	13	4	2	0	0
O	14	4	1	3	0
P	12	3	2	0	0

Table 8-3: Number and type of evaluator corrections.

Sixteen critiques, labelled A through P, were reviewed. The first column gives a rough idea of the size of each critique in numbers of sentences. Sentences were sometimes pieced together from more than one Roundsman "comment", so at times an evaluator had more than one correction for a sentence. Column two shows how many *phrasing* changes were suggested for each critique. (A more detailed discussion of the types of corrections in each of columns two through five is provided in the text.) Column three shows how many times the evaluator disagreed with the *content* of a comment. Column four indicates how many times the evaluator noted a problem with the *style* of the critique. Finally, column five shows how often the evaluator felt that some important comment was *missing* from the critique. For example, the reviewer of critique K suggested 4 phrasing changes, disagreed with the content of 1 comment, found the critique style wanting in 1 instance and felt that there was 1 comment that should have been included in the critique but was not included.

frequency of content disagreements. The evaluator of critiques A-I tended to note missing comments more frequently than the other oncologist.

Disagreements About Phrasing: The suggested phrasing changes were predominantly complaints that the output did not use oncology terminology properly (see Table 8-1). For example, in critique K Roundsman referred to one or another "protocol" but the phrase should be "arm". An example of phrasing which the oncologists categorized as "vague and unclear" was Roundsman's use of "the first protocol" to refer to a previously-mentioned intervention. They suggested reiterating the full intervention name. To one evaluator, the phrase "standard of care" (used to mean "the treatment most commonly employed in this situation") carried a menacing legal connotation and he suggested changing that phrase to "the conservative approach". One evaluator felt strongly that all five-year results should be mentioned before ten-year results. This is an accepted style of writing in this particular domain and deviating from this style appeared to interfere with communication to a significant degree.

Disagreements About Content: The extent of disagreement about content did not necessarily reflect how difficult the problem would be to fix. For example, in critique F the oncologist noted that a comment ending with "...institutions in the U.S." should have ended with "...institutions in the U.S. and Canada". This text-string error, which seems minor from the system-builder's point of view, was judged as "severe" (see Table 8-1) because it would be highly objectionable to the Canadian investigators who spent years participating in the study. A content disagreement which is more serious from a system-builder's point of view occurred in critique N, where a single comment about a mismatch was noted to be mixing together (and should not have been) two distinct clinical issues: non-uniformity of the surgical procedure and the use of a radiation "boost" in addition to the standard irradiation dose. In critiques G and H the oncologist disagreed with Roundsman's conclusion that the study could be used as support for viewing the two treatment approaches as equivalent. The oncologist felt that the mismatches between the study and the user's clinical problem were too great and that the study results could not confidently be used in the context under discussion.

Disagreements About Style: The most common objection to the style of the critique was that the oncologists wanted the first paragraph to include the clinical details which would be the subject of analysis in subsequent paragraphs. For example, if a mismatch was based upon the patient being pre-menopausal, they wanted the first paragraph to refer to "...122 pre-menopausal subjects..." rather than "122 subjects...". (This style of presentation is similar to the accepted style of presenting a history and physical on rounds: any clinical details which will become important in the analysis are mentioned in the factual portion of the presentation.) The other common complaint about the style was that the last paragraph was poorly formed: it did not have a good topic sentence to orient the reader to what was going to be said, it did not state the basis for its conclusions in enough detail, and the order of presentation was not optimal. As mentioned above, one of the two oncologists was much more interested in style issues than the other. After making "corrections" to a set of Roundsman's critiques, he outlined an abstract presentation style he would prefer for each paragraph. It is a perhaps a tribute to Roundsman that the oncologist was soon comparing the program output to his own writing, and making "editorial" suggestions as one might do for another writer.

Missing Comments: The oncologist felt that there were comments missing in critique B when radiation was mentioned: they wanted to also know the dosage and field of exposure. Another example of a missing comment occurred in critique E when the program used a study which had not included radiation to make inferences about a treatment plan which did include radiation: Roundsman made no mention of that mismatch issue. In critique A Roundsman mentioned that Amalric82 reported on a group of *pooled* stage I and stage II patients. The evaluator wanted to know more: was that all that the actual publication provided, or was there some data on how many patients were in each group? The same issue arose in his evaluation of critique C. One evaluator wanted all critiques to tell him not only what transpired in the clinical experiment but what research question(s) the investigators were asking, and what those investigators thought the results showed. In several critiques the evaluators felt that the last paragraph did not explicitly mention the user's proposed therapy, i.e., that this concluding paragraph did not return to the user's problem directly enough.

8.9.4. Discussion

The evaluation forms asked the oncologists to specify when they disliked something. It is important to say that they were, in general, pleased with the program's performance. In many cases the oncologist read entire paragraphs without objection, or commented that the points made by Roundsman were good ones. In particular, they felt that the kinds of mismatch comments which were being made were appropriate and critical to an intelligent appraisal of the studies. It was their feeling that the critiques would be significantly stronger with improvements in the stylistic organization and the phrasing. They found the approach to choice (the fourth paragraph in each critique) a reasonable one which reflected the "conservative" nature of breast cancer treatment: reluctance to deviate from the most commonly used treatment *unless* the study provided strong support for freedom to deviate.

In several instances the oncologist disagreed with the content of the critique but when the facts of the case were looked up it turned out that Roundsman was correct and the oncologist's memory was not completely accurate. For example, one oncologist was certain that the sample sizes given in critique F (a recent trial with which the oncologist was very familiar) were much larger than the actual sample sizes in the study. It was necessary to pull the actual publication from his files, search through the charts and tables to identify the subset under discussion, and finally to confirm that Roundsman's critique was correct. In critique J the oncologist disagreed with the critique's comment that the study subjects were all post-menopausal. The study in question is a well-known and controversial study and he felt that if they had been post-menopausal he would have remembered that aspect. In fact, the study subjects were all over 50 years of age (a criteria which is often used as defining post-menopausal). Thus, even for recent and well-known studies, the oncologists found that details of the study might be recalled more accurately by Roundsman.

What can be said about the *source* of the problems noted by the evaluators?

Source 1: Following the numbering in Table 8-4, the evaluation was very useful in bringing to light problems traceable to source 1-b. For example, the "nonstandard-intervention" component of the distance taxonomy should be *refined* further to include descendent nodes "nonuniform-intervention-procedure" and "intervention-slightly-different-from-common-approach" (these were detected in the evaluation of critique D). The evaluation of critique O pointed out that the "nonstandard-intervention" component was being used imprecisely to express what should be an *additional taxonomy component*: "endpoint-definition-misleading". The evaluator's review of critique N pointed out that one distance metric component was being used to represent two clinical issues which should not be mixed together. Evaluation of critique J made clear the need for changes to distance-estimators and the need for additional distance-estimators. For example, the year of critique J was 1977, yet it displayed knowledge that chemotherapy benefits pre-menopausal women (which was not really known until the early 1980's). Consequently the year in which that distance-estimator is added to the system must be later than 1977. It was known as early as 1972 however, that post-menopausal women have a different prognosis than pre-menopausal women *regardless* of treatment approach. This issue was missing from critique J because there is currently no distance-estimator in Roundsman to handle that issue. Minimal attention to source 1-b would provide additional detail to comments like "pooled stage I and II". In order for Roundsman to insert concise clinical descriptors into the first paragraph, distance metric components would have to be able to carry these descriptors (source 1-a).

Source 2: The implementation of the choice model (item 2-b in Table 8-4) should keep track more explicitly of the intermediate steps in making a choice. These

Possible Problem Sources

1. Distance metric
   a. Limitations of the model
   b. Limitations of the implementation

2. Choice and explanation
   a. Limitations of the model (multiattribute strategies)
   b. Limitations of the implementation

3. Text generation
   a. Limitations of the model (TEXTNET)
   b. Limitations of the implementation (i.e., problem could be rectified by altering prose-arcs and prose-states in particular nets *without* changes in the TEXTNET model).

4. Control functions (search of library, selection of stratum, identification of comparison objects.)

5. Interactions between studies

6. Knowledge representation for studies (comparisons, strata, interventions).

Table 8-4: Possible sources of problems with output.

intermediate steps could then provide more detailed justification in the final paragraph. In addition, there were two situations in which Roundsman stated that the total mismatches were minimal enough that the study could be used for the case under consideration; the oncologist disagreed and felt that the mismatches were too severe to use the study results. This is due to certain criteria in the implementation of the choice model which allow three serious mismatches before the study is deemed "too far away" from the clinical context to be used. This problem caused the oncologist to disagree with Roundsman's conclusion in the final paragraph. The implementation should make finer distinctions concerning the size and number of mismatches: when one mismatch is extremely large, it should count as more than one of the three "serious" mismatches. The "grain-size" available in the calibration of distance metric components (source 1-b) is adequate for a better solution, but the implementation of the choice model did not use that calibration to its full potential.

Source 3: Item 3-b (Table 8-4) was the source of many style and phrasing problems noted by the oncologists. For example, it would be possible enrich the text networks which produce the first paragraph so that Roundsman mentions those clinical details which are going to be the major elements of discussion in the second or third paragraphs. In addition, the nets currently used in Roundsman could be altered to reiterate the full names of the interventions rather than referring to them as "the second protocol". Minor work on item 3-b could also improve topic sentences and bring vocabulary in line with accepted oncology terminology.

Source 4: The most serious of the control function inadequacies (item 4 in Table 8-4) manifested itself in critique F: when certain patient information is not known at the time of the consultation (and *is* expected to be known at a later point in the course of treatment), but that information was a stratification criterion in the study, Roundsman selects the "closest" stratum and does the best it can with those results. The oncologist would prefer that the program examine both strata in the study and proceed to do parallel analyses, prefacing its discussion with "If the patient turns out to have condition X, then ..." and another section beginning "On the other hand, if the patient turns out to have condition Y, then...". This manner of critiquing would require significant alteration to the current control functions in Roundsman, although the representation for *studies* (comparison objects, strata, and distance metric knowledge) is robust enough to handle this new demand. Another problem, noted in critique O, also resulted from a control function inadequacy: when analyzing a three-arm study, Roundsman did not select the two most appropriate arms for analysis. Correction of this would require small changes to the control functions.

Source 5: Item 5 in Table 8-4 was not really formally evaluated: the oncologists were aware that the studies were being critiqued serially, without considering them in concert, and as a result they did not focus on that issue. A "missing comment" in critique L did, however, stem from this inter-study source. Critique L discussed a case-series report and the oncologist felt that the critique would be greatly strengthened if it made reference to the results of another study to say that the (series) results were comparable to results from a large study of another treatment approach. As discussed in Chapter 6, representing and making use of interactions between studies is a major issue which is a promising area for future research.

Source 6: would need attention in order to fill in certain comments noted as "missing" (as mentioned below in the summary) but it was not the cause of many problems.

Summary:

1. Correct *phrasing and style* are critical to the quality of the critique. (The two oncologists had different "thresholds" for being bothered by phrasing and style, but were in agreement that it was a critical issue in performance.) While phrasing might seem to system-builders to be a peripheral concern, the evaluation reinforces a point made by previous investigators [Teach 81] in medical informatics: the ability of the system to communicate in a style which is natural to the end-users is crucial to whether the system will be integrated into their decision-making activities. Fortunately this issue was appreciated in the early stages of this research (although somewhat forgotten as questions about knowledge representation and inference took center stage), so that Roundsman's TEXTNET facility was developed. The relative independence of text generation from the rest of the system allows us to make many improvements in the style and phrasing without any changes in Roundsman's control structure or knowledge base of studies.

   Most phrase and style alterations can be accomplished by changing the implemented text networks (source 3-b in Table 8-4). None of the disagreements about style and phrasing suggested that the TEXTNET model (source 3-a) was inadequate. When the phrase needing alteration is part of the study knowledge base (e.g., the value of the "specifics" slot in a distance metric component, which is source 1-b) then the system-builder must change the phrase within the knowledge base (examining the relevant text network to make sure that connecting phrases in the network still fit with the new phrase). This requires attention, but is quite manageable with TEXTNET. Addition of a one-word clinical descriptor to distance metric components (source 1-a) plus changes to text networks (source 3-b) would allow the first paragraph to mention clinical details which are going to be prominent issues in the second and third paragraphs.

2. Certain features of reasoning from empirical evidence in the clinical literature are *missing* from the current critiques, such as the capability to mention other studies as reinforcing or contradictory evidence and the use of other study results to "explain" aspects of the study under consideration. Interactions between studies, a major research topic, would have to be squarely addressed before case-series reports could compare their results to some external results. (See Chapter 6 for a fuller discussion of interactions between studies.) Referring again to Table 8-4, a moderate amount of change to source 6 would probably allow the system to be add comments specifying radiation dose and field, what

questions the investigators were asking and what they concluded. Minor changes to source 3-b would allow the last paragraph to add explicit references to the user's plan (which the evaluators noted as "missing comments"). Small changes to source 1-b would allow the system to add precision to comments like "a group of pooled stage I and II patients".

3. The *disagreements about content* point to sources 1-b, 2-b and 4. Refinement of the distance metric taxonomy (source 1-b) is "upward-compatible" with the existing taxonomy and consistent with the distance metric model. Other content problems require attention to the way in which Roundsman "sums up" a group of mismatches (source 2-b). The grain-size of the distance metric component calibration ("small", "medium" etc.) is adequate for an implementation which would do a much better job of "summing up" mismatches. Source 4 was responsible for the problem of Roundsman selecting the wrong study arms to use in its analysis. Finally, some disagreements about content stem from the variability inherent in clinical practice. Physicians may view the seriousness of mismatches differently, and they may feel differently about the strength of experimental evidence in support of a new treatment modality. Clearly, the advice of systems designed for clinical use must acknowledge the legitimacy of practice variability.

Chapter 9
Conclusions

9.1. Summary

In developing the prototype Roundsman system described in the previous chapters, we are exploring the proposition that the clinical literature can, and should, play a central role in computer-based decision support. Specifically, as discussed in the introduction to this book, the motivation underlying this research includes the following propositions:

- Reasoning from experimental evidence contained in the clinical literature is central to the decisions a physician makes in many areas of patient care. Medical artificial intelligence, heavily oriented toward *causal* modeling, has not adequately recognized this facet of medical reasoning.

- A computational model, based upon a declarative representation for published reports of clinical studies, can drive a computer program that selectively tailors knowledge of the clinical literature as it applies to a particular case.

- The development of such a computational model is an important first step toward filling a void in computer-based decision support systems. Furthermore, the model may help us better understand the general principles of reasoning from experimental evidence both in medicine and in other appropriate domains. This research therefore provides a base for further explicit analysis of these principles.

The Roundsman project delineates an explicit, computational model of medical decision-making which uses a structured representation of the clinical literature, together with a distance metric, to dynamically assess the "distance" between studies and a particular patient and treatment plan. Roundsman's knowledge representation derives from informal protocol analysis of experienced clinicians. The prose output generated by the model's computer implementation approximates target "scripts" of clinical reasoning developed in collaboration with an expert oncologist.

The impact of this research will be in four general areas:

1. Clinical practice: Physicians realize the very direct and crucial role the

clinical literature plays in helping them optimize their medical practice. The Roundsman system is a first step in exploring how the computer can help to bring a critical analysis of the relevant literature to the physician, structured around a particular patient and treatment decision.

2. Artificial Intelligence: The knowledge representation issues explored in reasoning from experimental evidence represent a challenge and an opportunity. Medicine and the social sciences will repeatedly present problem domains for which there are no reliable causal models, and in which reasoning from experimental evidence may be pivotal to problem-solving. System designers will therefore find it useful to investigate how practitioners reason from the empirical evidence. This reasoning process may well have a structure more complex than the *heuristic rules* which supported first-generation expert systems, and also quite unlike the *causal models* of more recent AI research. The Roundsman project models one such domain (the clinical literature) and it is hoped that this model will help researchers investigate other domains where decision-making relies on an understanding of experimental evidence.

3. Decision analysis: Decision analysis uses an axiom-based approach to decision-making which often helps clarify which data and value judgments have the largest effect on a particular decision. Computer systems have been built to assist users in framing their problem in decision-theoretic terms so that decision analytic techniques can then be applied. A central aspect of medical decision analysis is estimating the probability of events. This task demands a strong clinical background and experience reading biostatistical reports. Although this task is common to a range of decision analysis methodologies, there has been little explicit analysis of the reasoning process by which probabilities are assigned, and (to our knowledge) no attempts to develop a computational model of this process. The Roundsman project draws upon artificial intelligence techniques to develop a computational model which may therefore contribute to the theoretic base of medical decision analysis.

   There might well be advantages to interfacing a system like Roundsman to a decision-analytic system. This would combine the analytic capabilities of decision theory with Roundsman's ability to search a knowledge base of clinical literature and make assessments tailored to a particular patient and a specific intervention.

4. Bibliographic retrieval: Physicians seldom formalize their decisions to the

extent that decision analysis requires. Nevertheless, they use bibliographic retrieval systems analogously to the way in which decision analysts search the literature. The Roundsman system is a step toward the development of bibliographic retrieval systems which can make inferences about how well an article applies to the particular clinical problem facing the physician.

9.2. Limitations

The current Roundsman system focusses on a central and important component of the management of breast cancer. This model allows us to explore the design issues involved in reasoning from the literature. Roundsman's knowledge of breast cancer management is, however, hardly complete.

1. Roundsman does not currently include studies on chemotherapy. This limits the clinical applicability of Roundsman in contemporary breast cancer treatment. Chemotherapy is a rapidly-changing area of breast cancer management and has already shown a capability to cure certain types of breast cancer. Drug combinations are numerous and changing. They have serious side effects (e.g, sterility) which introduce "trade-off" issues into management. Physicians rely heavily on the clinical literature to provide the latest information on which patient groups do well on what drugs. As a result, the area of chemotherapy would lend itself well to Roundsman's type of analysis.

2. This research explores the process of reasoning from experimental evidence contained in the clinical literature. The heuristics of clinical practice were not the research focus and consequently Roundsman is unaware of some practical clinical issues. For example, breast cancer patients who present with coexisting heart disease, previous cancers or diabetes are treated in practice in a way which accommodates these other diseases. Although Roundsman might alert the user to the fact that a study did not include diabetic patients, it does not currently draw upon practical heuristics in order to accommodate the patient as an experienced clinician would do. Thus the scope of Roundsman's clinical knowledge was deliberately kept constrained to allow us to focus on the design issues involved.

3. The implementation of Roundsman's model of choice and explanation is limited. As mentioned in section 8.9, the implementation should make finer distinctions concerning the size and number of mismatches: when one mismatch is extremely large, it should count as more than one of the

three "serious" mismatches. The grain-size available in the calibration of distance metric components can support a better solution than the current implementation.

4. What would it entail to develop a system like Roundsman in other domains? Roundsman's distance metric model generalizes to other medical domains with the caveat that the model handles only a subset of all types of biomedical reports (see Table 2-1). Certainly the data structures (and hierarchies) representing *treatments* and *outcomes* would have to be redone to accommodate the new domain. In addition, the text networks would have to be re-implemented, using the unaltered TEXTNET model. Chapter 5 deliberately examines the applicability of the model of choice and explanation to other domains. Different domains highlight different features of the model. The usefulness of this approach to choice and explanation depends more on the goals of the system than on the domain. For example, our approach would be less useful for an audience which wants to model the components of each decision-making problem in more exact detail (e.g., assessing personal utilities for each outcome and looking at the expected-value of the overall decision). As will be mentioned in the next section, applying the Roundsman model to other domains is a promising area for future research.

5. Maintenance of the knowledge base over time is a challenging research issue which the current system does not address. The crux of the problem is interactions between studies as the knowledge base is updated; this promising area for future research is discussed at length in section 6.1.

9.3. Promising Areas for Extending the Research

Updating of the knowledge base

The development of sophisticated approaches to automatically update Roundsman's knowledge base is one of the most promising directions for future research. As discussed in Chapter 6, adding new studies should involve much more than "filling in slots" of a pre-determined representation scheme. The unique characteristics of a research report often cast previous reports in a new light, altering their interpretation. This issue as not been fully explored in the current system.

Roundsman does not help the user "fit" new studies into its knowledge base. This would entail automatically assisting the user in entering a new study. Central to this process would be to help the user encode the *inter-study* relationships that arise, as in the example described above. It is anticipated that the development of such a knowledge updating facility would be a vehicle to explore and clarify many aspects of reasoning from the empirical evidence in clinical literature which have not yet been uncovered in the Roundsman project.

Different medical domains

The character of breast cancer influences the research issues explored in the Roundsman project. For example, breast cancer is a life-threatening disease and the important studies concern the use of a treatment to prevent death. Since the prevention of death overrides most other concerns, this literature is not oriented toward studying all the minor morbidities of therapy - but these might emerge as central issues in a domain such as the drug treatment of arthritis or hypertension. (Arthritis medications can cause a patient to feel ill and can injure the kidney. Antihypertensive medications have a wide range of side effects.) In arthritis management, the clinician seeks to slow or halt progression of the disease while minimizing the unpleasant side effects of the drugs. It would be informative to develop a system like Roundsman in such a domain, and explore how the domain affects the system design.

Education

Physicians might use a system like Roundsman to generate a "review of the literature" for hypothetical cases or for cases being followed on rounds in a training hospital. This could be an interactive way of bringing students up-to-date about the latest clinical studies. This research direction might need a greater emphasis on user-modelling than in the current Roundsman system. The system would probably be able to teach more effectively if it knew what the physician's interests were, and how familiar the student already was with the state of knowledge in the domain.

Handling other classes of biomedical reports

Roundsman's studies are longitudinal studies of deliberate intervention. As Table 2-1 in Chapter 2 illustrates, there are several other classes of biomedical report. Roundsman's representational framework would adapt to *retrospective* studies of deliberate intervention, but *prospective observational* studies would stretch the limits of Roundsman's current knowledge representation. The studies in Roundsman are from an important class of biostatistical reports: comparison of treatments. Observational studies ask very different questions: What is the cause of disease? What is the incidence of disease? Exploring these and other classes of reports would address important clincial issues and would doubtless uncover new questions regarding knowledge representation.

This book contributes to the better understanding and development of fundamental models of medical decision making. The approach differs substantially from causal modeling in that there is no desire to model human pathophysiology, but rather to model the structure of experimental trials and their relevance to a physician's patient and treatment plan. The development of this computational model suggests a promising new direction for medical informatics; decision support systems which bring a critical analysis of the relevant literature to the physician, structured around a particular patient and treatment plan, might be a vital addition to the tools of practicing physicians. Furthermore, computational models of how physicians reason from the clinical literature may illuminate general principles of reasoning from experimental evidence, opening these principles up to further explicit analysis.

Appendix I
Internal Representation of the Studies in Roundsman's Library

This appendix outlines the internal representation of the twenty-four studies contained in the current Roundsman system. These studies are derived from actual publications in the clinical literature. The studies are built with the collaboration of an expert oncologist who has read the publications. In this appendix the studies are ordered chronologically and their contents are shown in a following format:

- Reference: a full reference for each publication can be found in the references section at the end of this book.

- Institution: location where the research was done.

- An enumeration of the *comparisons* contained in the study, as discussed more fully in Chapter 4. Shorthand descriptions of the two interventions are aligned in two columns, along with the sample size, endpoint measured and the proportion observed. the standard error of the difference between the proportions is recorded explicitly (if life-table analysis was used it may not be derivable from the proportions). These results were observed for a particular *stratum* which has an integer identifier.

- An enumeration of the *strata* contained in the study. These patient groups are defined by the values of clinical parameters. Parameter names are shown in lowercase on the left and parameter values are shown enclosed in parentheses on the right.

- A listing of the distance metric knowledge potentially used by Roundsman when assessing the study in the context of a particular patient and treatment plan. Each listed item is either (a) the name of a distance metric component or (b) a distance estimator. The integers listed after each item are the identifying numbers of *comparisons* which may use that distance metric component or distance estimator. The applicability of a methodological weakness does not in general depend on the clinical context and the use of a distance estimator; thus when a distance metric component is a methodological weakness, its name is simply listed. Distance-estimators are represented separately from studies. To reduce the system response-time, a portion of the distance assessment processing is done before run-time. That is, for each study, a search is made of all distance-estimators. Distance-estimators which are potentially useful in assessing the distance between the study and a clinical context (patient and plan) are identified, and an index of these distance-estimators is stored within the study.

[*In this appendix, explanatory text is italicized and enclosed in brackets.*]

Patey48

```
Reference: [Patey 48]
Institution: Middlesex Hospital, London

The COMPARISONS in Patey48:

1.  Radical-Mastectomy                     Tm-With-Axillary-Dissection
    18   patients                          18   patients
    OAS-3 = 0.78                           OAS-3 = 0.83
          standard error of the difference: 0.1318
          patient stratum concerned: 1

2.  Radical-Mastectomy                     Tm-With-Axillary-Dissection
    24   patients                          22   patients
    OAS-3 = 0.46                           OAS-3 = 0.45
          standard error of the difference: 0.14697
          patient stratum concerned: 2
```

[*Comparison 1 and 2 each concern radical mastectomy versus total mastectomy with axillary dissection. (Roundsman's treatment hierarchy is shown in Table 3-3.) The sample sizes and the proportions observed differ because the results concern different patient strata. In each comparison the endpoint measured was overall survival at three years (OAS-3). (Roundsman's outcome hierarchy is shown in Table 3-6.*]

```
The STRATA in Patey48:

1.  clinical stages:          (I II III)
    tumor sizes:              (UNKNOWN)
    clinical node staging:    (UNKNOWN)
    pathologic node staging:  (0)
    metastatic staging:       (MO)
    menopausal status:        (PRE POST)
    age-range:                (0 . 0)

2.  clinical stages:          (I II III)
    tumor sizes:              (UNKNOWN)
    clinical node staging:    (UNKNOWN)
```

```
pathologic node staging:  (1 2 3 4UP)
metastatic staging:       (MO)
menopausal status:        (PRE POST)
age-range:                (0 . 0)
```

[*The Patey48 publication described two strata, each of which included clincal stages I, II and III. One group of women had negative axillary nodes on pathologic exam and the other had positive nodes. Consequently, Roundsman's representation for strata 1 and 2 (above) each include clincal stages I, II and III but differ on pathologic node staging. Each stratum includes both pre- and post-menopausal women and no information is given about their age-range (default values shown for lower and upper bound ages).*]

```
The DISTANCE METRIC KNOWLEDGE in Patey48:

    Representative-Selection: 1 2
       se-change: DECREASE-SMALL
    Temporal-Drift: 1 2
       se-change: INCREASE-MODERATE
    Narrow-Stratum: 1 2
       se-change: DECREASE-SMALL
    Parallel-Non-Randomized-Controls: 1 2
       se-change: INCREASE-SMALL
    distance-estimator #20: 1
       dp-change: TOWARD-ZERO-MODERATE
    distance-estimator #21: 2
       dp-change: AWAY-FROM-ZERO-MODERATE
```

[*The first four items listed are methodological weaknesses, each of which pertains to comparisons 1 and 2. Distance-estimator #20 (represented separately from Patey48) has been identified as being potentially useful to comparison 1. Distance-estimator #21 has been identified as being potentially useful to comparison 2. The slots "dp-change" and "se-change" are described in Chapter 4.*]

McWhirter55

```
Reference: [McWhirter 55]
Institution: Edinburgh

The COMPARISONS in McWhirter55:

1.  Total-Mastectomy                      Intervention-External-To-Study
    Adjuvant-Radiation-Tx
    810  patients                         NIL
    OAS-5 = 0.6                           NIL
          standard error of the difference: 0
          patient stratum concerned: 1
```

[The sole comparison in McWhirter55 represents the results of a case series report on total mastectomy and adjuvant radiotherapy. There are no internal controls and the results must be compared to an intervention external to McWhirter55.]

```
The STRATA in McWhirter55:

1.  clinical stages:           (I II)
    tumor sizes:               (UNKNOWN)
    clinical node staging:     (UNKNOWN)
    pathologic node staging:   (UNKNOWN)
    metastatic staging:        (MO)
    menopausal status:         (PRE POST)
    age-range:                 (0 . 0)

The DISTANCE METRIC KNOWLEDGE in McWhirter55:

    External-Controls: 1
       se-change: INCREASE-MODERATE
    Wide-Stratum: 1
       se-change: INCREASE-MODERATE
    distance-estimator #24
       se-change: INCREASE-EXTREME
    Nonstandard-Stage: 1
       se-change: INCREASE-SMALL
```

Haagensen63

```
Reference: [Haagensen 63]
Institution: Columbia-Presbyterian, New York

The COMPARISONS in Haagensen63:

1.  Radical-Mastectomy                Intervention-External-To-Study
    Adjuvant-Radiation-Tx
    344  patients                     NIL
    OAS-5 = 0.85                      NIL
          standard error of the difference: 0
          patient stratum concerned: 1

2.  Radical-Mastectomy                Intervention-External-To-Study
    Adjuvant-Radiation-Tx
    138  patients                     NIL
    OAS-5 = 0.59                      NIL
          standard error of the difference: 0
          patient stratum concerned: 2

The STRATA in Haagensen63:

1.  clinical stages:           (I II III)
    tumor sizes:               (T1A T2A T3A)
    clinical node staging:     (NO N1A)
    pathologic node staging:   (UNKNOWN)
```

```
    metastatic staging:       (M0)
    menopausal status:        (PRE POST)
    age-range:                (20 . 80)

2.  clinical stages:          (I II III)
    tumor sizes:              (T1A T2A T3A)
    clinical node staging:    (N1B)
    pathologic node staging:  (UNKNOWN)
    metastatic staging:       (M0)
    menopausal status:        (PRE POST)
    age-range:                (20 . 80)
```

The DISTANCE METRIC KNOWLEDGE in Haagensen63:

```
    Highly-Reliable-Author: 1 2
       se-change: DECREASE-SMALL
    Long-Accrual-Period: 1 2
       se-change: INCREASE-SMALL
    Authors-Conclusions-Strong: 1 2
    External-Controls: 1 2
       se-change: INCREASE-SMALL
    Nonstandard-Intervention: 1 2
       se-change: NEGLIGIBLE
    Nonstandard-Intervention: 1 2
       se-change: NEGLIGIBLE
    distance-estimator #11: 1
       se-change: NONE
    distance-estimator #10: 1
       dp-change: NONE
    distance-estimator #4: 2
       se-change: NONE
```

Handley63

Reference: [Handley 63]
Institution: Middlesex Hospital, London

The COMPARISONS in Handley63:

```
1.  Tm-With-Axillary-Dissection       Intervention-External-To-Study
    Adjuvant-Radiation-Tx
    77   patients                     0    patients
    OAS-5 = 0.75                      NIL
          standard error of the difference: 0
          patient stratum concerned: 1

2.  Tm-With-Axillary-Dissection       Intervention-External-To-Study
    Adjuvant-Radiation-Tx
    58   patients                     0    patients
    OAS-5 = 0.57                      NIL
          standard error of the difference: 0
          patient stratum concerned: 2
```

The STRATA in Handley63:

```
1.  clinical stages:            (I II III)
    tumor sizes:                (T1A T2A T3A)
    clinical node staging:      (N0 N1A)
    pathologic node staging:    (UNKNOWN)
    metastatic staging:         (M0)
    menopausal status:          (PRE POST)
    age-range:                  (20 . 80)

2.  clinical stages:            (I II III)
    tumor sizes:                (T1A T2A T3A)
    clinical node staging:      (N1B)
    pathologic node staging:    (UNKNOWN)
    metastatic staging:         (M0)
    menopausal status:          (PRE POST)
    age-range:                  (20 . 80)
```

```
The DISTANCE METRIC KNOWLEDGE in Handley63:

    Selection-Bias: 1 2
       se-change: INCREASE-MODERATE
    External-Controls: 1 2
       se-change: INCREASE-MODERATE
    Nonstandard-Intervention: 1 2
       se-change: NEGLIGIBLE
    distance-estimator #
       dp-change: TOWARD-ZERO-SMALL
    distance-estimator #11: 1
       se-change: NONE
    distance-estimator #10: 1
       dp-change: NONE
    distance-estimator #4: 2
       se-change: NONE
```

Kaee65

```
Reference: [Kaee 65]
Institution: Copenhagen

The COMPARISONS in kaee65:

1.  Adjuvant-Radiation-Tx                Radical-Mastectomy
    Total-Mastectomy
    70  patients                         65  patients
    OAS-5 = 0.46                         OAS-5 = 0.46
          standard error of the difference: 0.08585
          patient stratum concerned: 2

2.  Adjuvant-Radiation-Tx                Radical-Mastectomy
    Total-Mastectomy
    149  patients                        141  patients
    OAS-5 = 0.67                         OAS-5 = 0.68
          standard error of the difference: 0.05502
          patient stratum concerned: 1
```

```
3.  Adjuvant-Radiation-Tx              Radical-Mastectomy
    Total-Mastectomy
    70   patients                      65   patients
    RFS-5 = 0.36                       RFS-5 = 0.37
          standard error of the difference: 0.08293
          patient stratum concerned: 2

4.  Adjuvant-Radiation-Tx              Radical-Mastectomy
    Total-Mastectomy
    149  patients                      141  patients
    RFS-5 = 0.67                       RFS-5 = 0.68
          standard error of the difference: 0.05502
          patient stratum concerned: 1


The STRATA in kaee65:

1.  clinical stages:           (I)
    tumor sizes:               (UNKNOWN)
    clinical node staging:     (UNKNOWN)
    pathologic node staging:   (UNKNOWN)
    metastatic staging:        (M0)
    menopausal status:         (PRE POST)
    age-range:                 (20 . 80)

2.  clinical stages:           (II)
    tumor sizes:               (UNKNOWN)
    clinical node staging:     (UNKNOWN)
    pathologic node staging:   (UNKNOWN)
    metastatic staging:        (M0)
    menopausal status:         (PRE POST)
    age-range:                 (20 . 80)


The DISTANCE METRIC KNOWLEDGE in kaee65:

    Authors-Conclusions-Strong: 1 2 3 4
    Parallel-Randomized-Controls: 1 2 3 4
       se-change: DECREASE-SMALL
    Large-Number-Of-Exclusions: 1 2 3 4
       se-change: INCREASE-SMALL
    Selection-Bias: 1 3
       dp-change: NEGATIVE-SMALL
    Possibly-Confounding-Intervention-Variable: 1 2 3 4
       se-change: INCREASE-SMALL
    distance-estimator #24: 1 2 3 4
       se-change: INCREASE-EXTREME
    Nonstandard-Intervention: 1 2 3 4
       dp-change: NEGLIGIBLE
    distance-estimator #
       dp-change: NEGLIGIBLE
    distance-estimator #8: 1 3
       dp-change: TOWARD-ZERO-MODERATE
    distance-estimator #4: 1 3
       se-change: NONE
    distance-estimator #6: 2 4
       dp-change: AWAY-FROM-ZERO-MODERATE
    distance-estimator #5: 2 4
```

```
        se-change: NONE
```

Brinkley66

```
Reference: [Brinkley 66]
Institution: Addenbrooke's Hospital Cambridge

The COMPARISONS in Brinkley66:

1.  Radical-Mastectomy                  Tm-With-Axillary-Dissection
    Adjuvant-Radiation-Tx               Adjuvant-Radiation-Tx
    91   patients                       113  patients
    RFS-5 = 0.51                        RFS-5 = 0.58
          standard error of the difference: 0.08147
          patient stratum concerned: 1

2.  Radical-Mastectomy                  Tm-With-Axillary-Dissection
    Adjuvant-Radiation-Tx               Adjuvant-Radiation-Tx
    91   patients                       113  patients
    OAS-5 = 0.54                        OAS-5 = 0.66
          standard error of the difference: 0.08797
          patient stratum concerned: 1


The STRATA in Brinkley66:

1.  clinical stages:             (II)
    tumor sizes:                 (UNKNOWN)
    clinical node staging:       (UNKNOWN)
    pathologic node staging:     (UNKNOWN)
    metastatic staging:          (M0)
    menopausal status:           (PRE POST)
    age-range:                   (20 . 80)


The DISTANCE METRIC KNOWLEDGE in Brinkley66:

    Parallel-Randomized-Controls: 1 2
       se-change: DECREASE-SMALL
    Good-Analysis-Of-Confounding-Variables: 1 2
       se-change: DECREASE-SMALL
    Narrow-Stratum: 1 2
       se-change: DECREASE-SMALL
    distance-estimator #8: 1 2
       dp-change: TOWARD-ZERO-MODERATE
    distance-estimator #4: 1 2
       se-change: NONE
```

Peters67

```
Reference: [Peters 67]
Institution: Princess Margaret Hospital, Toronto

The COMPARISONS in peters67:
```

```
1.  Radical-Mastectomy                 Wide-Excision
    Adjuvant-Radiation-Tx              Adjuvant-Radiation-Tx
    247  patients                      94   patients
    OAS-5 = 0.72                       OAS-5 = 0.76
          standard error of the difference: 0.05021
          patient stratum concerned: 1
```

```
The STRATA in peters67:

1.  clinical stages:            (I II)
    tumor sizes:                (T1A T2A)
    clinical node staging:      (N0 N1A)
    pathologic node staging:    (UNKNOWN)
    metastatic staging:         (M0)
    menopausal status:          (PRE POST)
    age-range:                  (20 . 80)
```

```
The DISTANCE METRIC KNOWLEDGE in peters67:

    Wide-Stratum: 1
       se-change: INCREASE-SMALL
    Long-Accrual-Period: 1
       se-change: INCREASE-MODERATE
    Parallel-Non-Randomized-Controls: 1
       se-change: INCREASE-MODERATE
    Modality-Slightly-Dissimilar: 1
       se-change: NEGLIGIBLE
    distance-estimator #19: 1
       dp-change: AWAY-FROM-ZERO-SMALL
    distance-estimator #18: 1
       dp-change: TOWARD-ZERO-SMALL
```

Handley69

```
Reference: [Handley 69]
Institution: Middlesex Hospital, London

The COMPARISONS in Handley69:

1.  Tm-With-Axillary-Dissection       Intervention-External-To-Study
    Adjuvant-Radiation-Tx
    77   patients                     0    patients
    OAS-5 = 0.75                      NIL
          standard error of the difference: 0
          patient stratum concerned: 1

2.  Tm-With-Axillary-Dissection       Intervention-External-To-Study
    Adjuvant-Radiation-Tx
    58   patients                     NIL
    OAS-5 = 0.57                      NIL
          standard error of the difference: 0
          patient stratum concerned: 2

3.  Tm-With-Axillary-Dissection       Intervention-External-To-Study
```

```
    Adjuvant-Radiation-Tx
    77   patients                       0    patients
    OAS-10 = 0.61                       NIL
          standard error of the difference: 0
          patient stratum concerned: 1

4.  Tm-With-Axillary-Dissection         Intervention-External-To-Study
    Adjuvant-Radiation-Tx
    58   patients                       NIL
    OAS-10 = 0.25                       NIL
          standard error of the difference: 0
          patient stratum concerned: 2

5.  Tm-With-Axillary-Dissection         Intervention-External-To-Study
    Adjuvant-Radiation-Tx
    77   patients                       NIL
    LRRF-10 = 0.84                      NIL
          standard error of the difference: 0
          patient stratum concerned: 1

6.  Tm-With-Axillary-Dissection         Intervention-External-To-Study
    Adjuvant-Radiation-Tx
    58   patients                       NIL
    LRRF-10 = 0.74                      NIL
          standard error of the difference: 0
          patient stratum concerned: 2


The STRATA in Handley69:

1.  clinical stages:            (I II III)
    tumor sizes:                (T1A T2A T3A)
    clinical node staging:      (N0 N1A)
    pathologic node staging:    (UNKNOWN)
    metastatic staging:         (M0)
    menopausal status:          (PRE POST)
    age-range:                  (20 . 80)

2.  clinical stages:            (I II III)
    tumor sizes:                (T1A T2A T3A)
    clinical node staging:      (N1B)
    pathologic node staging:    (UNKNOWN)
    metastatic staging:         (M0)
    menopausal status:          (PRE POST)
    age-range:                  (20 . 80)


The DISTANCE METRIC KNOWLEDGE in Handley69:

    Selection-Bias: 1 2 3 4 5 6
       se-change: INCREASE-MODERATE
    External-Controls: 1 2 3 4 5 6
       se-change: INCREASE-MODERATE
    Nonstandard-Intervention: 1 2 3 4 5 6
       se-change: NEGLIGIBLE
    distance-estimator #
       dp-change: TOWARD-ZERO-SMALL
    distance-estimator #11: 1 3 5
```

```
   se-change: NONE
distance-estimator #10: 1 3 5
   dp-change: NONE
distance-estimator #4: 2 4 6
   se-change: NONE
```

Haagensen69

```
Reference: [Haagensen 69]
Institution: Columbia-Presbyterian, New York

The COMPARISONS in haagensen69:

1.  Radical-Mastectomy                Intervention-External-To-Study
    Adjuvant-Radiation-Tx
    344  patients                     NIL
    OAS-5 = 0.85                      NIL
          standard error of the difference: 0
          patient stratum concerned: 1

3.  Radical-Mastectomy                Intervention-External-To-Study
    Adjuvant-Radiation-Tx
    344  patients                     NIL
    OAS-10 = 0.69                     NIL
          standard error of the difference: 0
          patient stratum concerned: 1

2.  Radical-Mastectomy                Intervention-External-To-Study
    Adjuvant-Radiation-Tx
    138  patients                     NIL
    OAS-5 = 0.59                      NIL
          standard error of the difference: 0
          patient stratum concerned: 2

4.  Radical-Mastectomy                Intervention-External-To-Study
    Adjuvant-Radiation-Tx
    138  patients                     NIL
    OAS-5 = 0.37                      NIL
          standard error of the difference: 0
          patient stratum concerned: 2


The STRATA in haagensen69:

1.  clinical stages:            (I II III)
    tumor sizes:                (T1A T2A T3A)
    clinical node staging:      (NO N1A)
    pathologic node staging:    (UNKNOWN)
    metastatic staging:         (MO)
    menopausal status:          (PRE POST)
    age-range:                  (20 . 80)

2.  clinical stages:            (I II III)
    tumor sizes:                (T1A T2A T3A)
    clinical node staging:      (N1B)
    pathologic node staging:    (UNKNOWN)
```

```
metastatic staging:        (MO)
menopausal status:         (PRE POST)
age-range:                 (20 . 80)
```

```
The DISTANCE METRIC KNOWLEDGE in haagensen69:

    Highly-Reliable-Author: 1 3 2 4
       se-change: DECREASE-SMALL
    Long-Accrual-Period: 1 3 2 4
       se-change: INCREASE-SMALL
    Authors-Conclusions-Strong: 1 3 2 4
    External-Controls: 1 3 2 4
       se-change: INCREASE-SMALL
    Nonstandard-Intervention: 1 3 2 4
       se-change: NEGLIGIBLE
    Nonstandard-Intervention: 1 3 2 4
       se-change: NEGLIGIBLE
    distance-estimator #11: 1 3
       se-change: NONE
    distance-estimator #10: 1 3
       dp-change: NONE
    distance-estimator #4: 2 4
       se-change: NONE
```

Fisher70

```
Reference: [Fisher 70]
Institution: 25 participating hospitals and universities in the United

The COMPARISONS in Fisher70:

1.  Radical-Mastectomy                     Radical-Mastectomy
    Adjuvant-Radiation-Tx
    56   patients                          96   patients
    RFS-5 = 0.78                           RFS-5 = 0.76
          standard error of the difference: 0.07046
          patient stratum concerned: 1

2.  Radical-Mastectomy                     Radical-Mastectomy
    Adjuvant-Radiation-Tx
    124  patients                          139  patients
    RFS-5 = 0.38                           RFS-5 = 0.32
          standard error of the difference: 0.05887
          patient stratum concerned: 2

3.  Radical-Mastectomy                     Radical-Mastectomy
    Adjuvant-Radiation-Tx
    62   patients                          97   patients
    OAS-5 = 0.74                           OAS-5 = 0.79
          standard error of the difference: 0.06938
          patient stratum concerned: 1

4.  Radical-Mastectomy                     Radical-Mastectomy
    Adjuvant-Radiation-Tx
    133  patients                          136  patients
```

```
    OAS-5 = 0.47                         OAS-5 = 0.49
          standard error of the difference: 0.06091
          patient stratum concerned: 2

5.  Radical-Mastectomy                   Radical-Mastectomy
    Adjuvant-Radiation-Tx
    124  patients                        139  patients
    LRRFS-5 = 0.47                       LRRFS-5 = 0.58
          standard error of the difference: 0.06133
          patient stratum concerned: 2

6.  Radical-Mastectomy                   Radical-Mastectomy
    Adjuvant-Radiation-Tx
    56   patients                        96   patients
    LRRFS-5 = 0.88                       LRRFS-5 = 0.8
          standard error of the difference: 0.0596
          patient stratum concerned: 1


The STRATA in Fisher70:

1.  clinical stages:            (I II)
    tumor sizes:                (TO T1A T2A)
    clinical node staging:      (NO N1A N1B)
    pathologic node staging:    (0)
    metastatic staging:         (MO)
    menopausal status:          (PRE POST)
    age-range:                  (20 . 80)

2.  clinical stages:            (I II)
    tumor sizes:                (TO T1A T2A)
    clinical node staging:      (NO N1A N1B)
    pathologic node staging:    (1 2 3 4UP)
    metastatic staging:         (MO)
    menopausal status:          (PRE POST)
    age-range:                  (20 . 80)


The DISTANCE METRIC KNOWLEDGE in Fisher70:

    Large-Number-Of-Exclusions: 1 2 3 4 5 6
       se-change: INCREASE-MODERATE
    Parallel-Randomized-Controls: 1 2 3 4 5 6
       se-change: DECREASE-SMALL
    distance-estimator #20: 1 3 6
       dp-change: TOWARD-ZERO-MODERATE
    distance-estimator #21: 2 4 5
       dp-change: AWAY-FROM-ZERO-MODERATE
```

Brinkley71

```
Reference: [Brinkley 71]
Institution: Addenbrooke's Hospital Cambridge

The COMPARISONS in brinkley71:
```

```
1.  Radical-Mastectomy                   Tm-With-Axillary-Dissection
    Adjuvant-Radiation-Tx                Adjuvant-Radiation-Tx
    91  patients                         113  patients
    RFS-5 = 0.53                         RFS-5 = 0.58
          standard error of the difference: 0.07
          patient stratum concerned: 1

2.  Radical-Mastectomy                   Tm-With-Axillary-Dissection
    Adjuvant-Radiation-Tx                Adjuvant-Radiation-Tx
    91  patients                         113  patients
    OAS-10 = 0.49                        OAS-10 = 0.46
          standard error of the difference: 0.077
          patient stratum concerned: 1

3.  Radical-Mastectomy                   Tm-With-Axillary-Dissection
    Adjuvant-Radiation-Tx                Adjuvant-Radiation-Tx
    91  patients                         113  patients
    RFS-10 = 0.42                        RFS-10 = 0.46
          standard error of the difference: 0.074
          patient stratum concerned: 1
```

```
The STRATA in brinkley71:

1.  clinical stages:           (II)
    tumor sizes:               (UNKNOWN)
    clinical node staging:     (UNKNOWN)
    pathologic node staging:   (UNKNOWN)
    metastatic staging:        (M0)
    menopausal status:         (PRE POST)
    age-range:                 (20 . 80)
```

```
The DISTANCE METRIC KNOWLEDGE in brinkley71:

    Parallel-Randomized-Controls: 1 2 3
       se-change: DECREASE-SMALL
    Authors-Conclusions-Strong: 1 2 3
    Good-Analysis-Of-Confounding-Variables: 1 2 3
       se-change: DECREASE-SMALL
    Narrow-Stratum: 1 2 3
       se-change: DECREASE-SMALL
    distance-estimator #8: 1 2 3
       dp-change: TOWARD-ZERO-MODERATE
    distance-estimator #4: 1 2 3
       se-change: NONE
```

Atkins72

```
Reference: [Atkins 72]
Institution: Guy's Hospital, England

The COMPARISONS in Atkins72:

1.  Radical-Mastectomy                   Wide-Excision
    Adjuvant-Radiation-Tx                Adjuvant-Radiation-Tx
```

```
    108  patients                          112  patients
    OAS-5 = 0.8                            OAS-5 = 0.78
          standard error of the difference: 0.0549
          patient stratum concerned: 1

2.  Radical-Mastectomy                     Wide-Excision
    Adjuvant-Radiation-Tx                  Adjuvant-Radiation-Tx
    108  patients                          112  patients
    LRRF-5 = 0.92                          LRRF-5 = 0.8
          standard error of the difference: 0.04594
          patient stratum concerned: 1

3.  Radical-Mastectomy                     Wide-Excision
    Adjuvant-Radiation-Tx                  Adjuvant-Radiation-Tx
    80   patients                          70   patients
    OAS-5 = 0.72                           OAS-5 = 0.56
          standard error of the difference: 0.16
          patient stratum concerned: 2

4.  Radical-Mastectomy                     Wide-Excision
    Adjuvant-Radiation-Tx                  Adjuvant-Radiation-Tx
    80   patients                          70   patients
    LRRF-5 = 0.84                          LRRF-5 = 0.52
          standard error of the difference: 0.1
          patient stratum concerned: 2

5.  Radical-Mastectomy                     Wide-Excision
    Adjuvant-Radiation-Tx                  Adjuvant-Radiation-Tx
    80   patients                          70   patients
    OAS-10 = 0.58                          OAS-10 = 0.24
          standard error of the difference: 0.17
          patient stratum concerned: 2


The STRATA in Atkins72:

1.  clinical stages:           (I)
    tumor sizes:               (T0 T1A T1B)
    clinical node staging:     (N0 N1A)
    pathologic node staging:   (UNKNOWN)
    metastatic staging:        (M0)
    menopausal status:         (POST)
    age-range:                 (50 . 80)

2.  clinical stages:           (II)
    tumor sizes:               (T2A T2B)
    clinical node staging:     (N1B)
    pathologic node staging:   (UNKNOWN)
    metastatic staging:        (M0)
    menopausal status:         (POST)
    age-range:                 (50 . 80)


The DISTANCE METRIC KNOWLEDGE in Atkins72:

    Parallel-Randomized-Controls: 1 2 3 4 5
       se-change: DECREASE-SMALL
    Sketchy-Statistical-Reporting: 1 2 3 4 5
```

```
      se-change: INCREASE-SMALL
   Authors-Conclusions-Strong: 1 2 3 4 5
   distance-estimator #
      se-change: NEGLIGIBLE
   distance-estimator #
      dp-change: NEGATIVE-MODERATE
   distance-estimator #5: 1 2
      se-change: NONE
   distance-estimator #3: 1 2 3 4 5
      dp-change: NEGLIGIBLE
   distance-estimator #4: 3 4 5
      se-change: NONE
```

Fisher77

```
Reference: [Fisher 77]
Institution: 34 institutions in the U.S. and Canada

The COMPARISONS in fisher77:

4.  Total-Mastectomy                  Total-Mastectomy
    Adjuvant-Radiation-Tx
    352  patients                     365  patients
    RFS-3 = 0.75                      RFS-3 = 0.75
          standard error of the difference: 0.05833
          patient stratum concerned: 1

5.  Total-Mastectomy                  Total-Mastectomy
    Adjuvant-Radiation-Tx
    352  patients                     365  patients
    OAS-3 = 0.85                      OAS-3 = 0.85
          standard error of the difference: 0.04458
          patient stratum concerned: 1

6.  Radical-Mastectomy                Total-Mastectomy
                                      Adjuvant-Radiation-Tx
    362  patients                     352  patients
    RFS-3 = 0.75                      RFS-3 = 0.75
          standard error of the difference: 0.05662
          patient stratum concerned: 1

7.  Radical-Mastectomy                Total-Mastectomy
                                      Adjuvant-Radiation-Tx
    362  patients                     352  patients
    OAS-3 = 0.85                      OAS-3 = 0.85
          standard error of the difference: 0.04404
          patient stratum concerned: 1

8.  Radical-Mastectomy                Total-Mastectomy
    362  patients                     365  patients
    RFS-3 = 0.75                      RFS-3 = 0.75
          standard error of the difference: 0.05511
          patient stratum concerned: 1

9.  Radical-Mastectomy                Total-Mastectomy
    362  patients                     365  patients
```

```
    OAS-3 = 0.85                          OAS-3 = 0.85
          standard error of the difference: 0.04181
          patient stratum concerned: 1

11. Radical-Mastectomy                    Total-Mastectomy
                                          Adjuvant-Radiation-Tx
    292  patients                         294  patients
    RFS-3 = 0.6                           RFS-3 = 0.6
          standard error of the difference: 0.0877
          patient stratum concerned: 2

12. Radical-Mastectomy                    Total-Mastectomy
                                          Adjuvant-Radiation-Tx
    292  patients                         294  patients
    OAS-3 = 0.75                          OAS-3 = 0.75
          standard error of the difference: 0.06626
          patient stratum concerned: 2


The STRATA in fisher77:

1.  clinical stages:             (I II III)
    tumor sizes:                 (T1A T2A T3A)
    clinical node staging:       (NO N1A)
    pathologic node staging:     (UNKNOWN)
    metastatic staging:          (MO)
    menopausal status:           (PRE POST)
    age-range:                   (20 . 80)

2.  clinical stages:             (I II III)
    tumor sizes:                 (T1A T2A T3A)
    clinical node staging:       (N1B)
    pathologic node staging:     (UNKNOWN)
    metastatic staging:          (MO)
    menopausal status:           (PRE POST)
    age-range:                   (20 . 80)


The DISTANCE METRIC KNOWLEDGE in fisher77:

    Immature-Results: 4 5 6 7 8 9 11 12
       se-change: INCREASE-SMALL
    Parallel-Randomized-Controls: 4 5 6 7 8 9 11 12
       se-change: DECREASE-SMALL
    Sketchy-Statistical-Reporting: 4 5 6 7 8 9 11 12
       se-change: NEGLIGIBLE
    Highly-Reliable-Author: 4 5 6 7 8 9 11 12
       se-change: DECREASE-MODERATE
    Modification-Of-Intervention: 4 5 8 9
       se-change: NEGLIGIBLE
    distance-estimator #11: 4 5 6 7 8 9
       se-change: NONE
    distance-estimator #10: 4 5 6 7 8 9
       dp-change: NONE
    distance-estimator #9: 4 5 6 7 8 9
       dp-change: AWAY-FROM-ZERO-MODERATE
    distance-estimator #14: 11 12
       dp-change: TOWARD-ZERO-MODERATE
```

```
distance-estimator #13: 11 12
   dp-change: AWAY-FROM-ZERO-MODERATE
distance-estimator #12: 11 12
   dp-change: NONE
```

Hayward77

```
Reference: [Hayward 77]
Institution: Guy's Hospital, England

The COMPARISONS in hayward77:

1.  Radical-Mastectomy                  Wide-Excision
    Adjuvant-Radiation-Tx               Adjuvant-Radiation-Tx
    108  patients                       112  patients
    OAS-5 = 0.72                        OAS-5 = 0.71
          standard error of the difference: 0.06087
          patient stratum concerned: 1

2.  Radical-Mastectomy                  Wide-Excision
    Adjuvant-Radiation-Tx               Adjuvant-Radiation-Tx
    108  patients                       112  patients
    OAS-10 = 0.52                       OAS-10 = 0.58
          standard error of the difference: 0.09472
          patient stratum concerned: 1

3.  Radical-Mastectomy                  Wide-Excision
    Adjuvant-Radiation-Tx               Adjuvant-Radiation-Tx
    108  patients                       112  patients
    LRRF-5 = 0.89                       LRRF-5 = 0.75
          standard error of the difference: 0.0508
          patient stratum concerned: 1

4.  Radical-Mastectomy                  Wide-Excision
    Adjuvant-Radiation-Tx               Adjuvant-Radiation-Tx
    108  patients                       112  patients
    LRRF-10 = 0.85                      LRRF-10 = 0.63
          standard error of the difference: 0.08077
          patient stratum concerned: 1

5.  Radical-Mastectomy                  Wide-Excision
    Adjuvant-Radiation-Tx               Adjuvant-Radiation-Tx
    80   patients                       70   patients
    OAS-5 = 0.65                        OAS-5 = 0.6
          standard error of the difference: 0.0792
          patient stratum concerned: 2

6.  Radical-Mastectomy                  Wide-Excision
    Adjuvant-Radiation-Tx               Adjuvant-Radiation-Tx
    80   patients                       70   patients
    OAS-10 = 0.43                       OAS-10 = 0.3
          standard error of the difference: 0.11012
          patient stratum concerned: 2

7.  Radical-Mastectomy                  Wide-Excision
    Adjuvant-Radiation-Tx               Adjuvant-Radiation-Tx
```

```
    80   patients                        70   patients
    LRRF-5 = 0.79                        LRRF-5 = 0.43
         standard error of the difference: 0.07467
         patient stratum concerned: 2

8.  Radical-Mastectomy                   Wide-Excision
    Adjuvant-Radiation-Tx                Adjuvant-Radiation-Tx
    80   patients                        70   patients
    LRRF-10 = 0.65                       LRRF-10 = 0.43
         standard error of the difference: 0.11265
         patient stratum concerned: 2


The STRATA in hayward77:

1.  clinical stages:            (I)
    tumor sizes:                (T0 T1A T1B)
    clinical node staging:      (N0 N1A)
    pathologic node staging:    (UNKNOWN)
    metastatic staging:         (M0)
    menopausal status:          (POST)
    age-range:                  (50 . 80)

2.  clinical stages:            (II)
    tumor sizes:                (T2A T2B)
    clinical node staging:      (N1B)
    pathologic node staging:    (UNKNOWN)
    metastatic staging:         (M0)
    menopausal status:          (POST)
    age-range:                  (50 . 80)


The DISTANCE METRIC KNOWLEDGE in hayward77:

    Parallel-Randomized-Controls: 1 2 3 4 5 6 7 8
       se-change: DECREASE-SMALL
    Sketchy-Statistical-Reporting: 1 2 3 4 5 6 7 8
       se-change: INCREASE-SMALL
    Authors-Conclusions-Strong: 1 2 3 4 5 6 7 8
    distance-estimator #
       se-change: NEGLIGIBLE
    distance-estimator #
       dp-change: NEGATIVE-MODERATE
    distance-estimator #4: 1 2 3 4 5 6 7 8
       se-change: NONE
    distance-estimator #3: 1 2 3 4 5 6 7 8
       dp-change: NEGLIGIBLE
```

Levene77

```
Reference: [Levene 77]
Institution: the Joint Center for Radiation Therapy, Boston

The COMPARISONS in levene77:

1.  Wide-Excision                        Intervention-External-To-Study
```

```
    Adjuvant-Radiation-Tx
    19   patients                       NIL
    OAS-5 = 1.0                         NIL
          standard error of the difference: 0
          patient stratum concerned: 1

2.  Wide-Excision                       Intervention-External-To-Study
    Adjuvant-Radiation-Tx
    45   patients                       NIL
    OAS-5 = 0.65                        NIL
          standard error of the difference: 0
          patient stratum concerned: 2


The STRATA in levene77:

1.  clinical stages:            (I)
    tumor sizes:                (T0 T1A T1B)
    clinical node staging:      (N0 N1A)
    pathologic node staging:    (UNKNOWN)
    metastatic staging:         (M0)
    menopausal status:          (PRE POST)
    age-range:                  (20 . 80)

2.  clinical stages:            (II)
    tumor sizes:                (T2A T2B)
    clinical node staging:      (N1B)
    pathologic node staging:    (UNKNOWN)
    metastatic staging:         (M0)
    menopausal status:          (PRE POST)
    age-range:                  (20 . 80)


The DISTANCE METRIC KNOWLEDGE in levene77:

    Sketchy-Statistical-Reporting: 1 2
       se-change: INCREASE-SMALL
    Selection-Bias: 1 2
       se-change: INCREASE-MODERATE
    External-Controls: 1 2
       se-change: INCREASE-EXTREME
    Immature-Results: 1
       se-change: INCREASE-MODERATE
    Nonstandard-Outcome: 1 2
       se-change: INCREASE-MODERATE
    Immature-Results: 2
       se-change: INCREASE-MODERATE
    Nonstandard-Intervention: 1 2
       se-change: INCREASE-SMALL
    distance-estimator #5: 1
       se-change: NONE
    distance-estimator #4: 2
       se-change: NONE
```

Peters77

```
Reference: [Peters 77]
Institution: Princess Margaret Hospital, Toronto

The COMPARISONS in peters77:

1.  Wide-Excision                      Radical-Mastectomy
    Adjuvant-Radiation-Tx              Adjuvant-Radiation-Tx
    203  patients                      609  patients
    OAS-10 = 0.75                      OAS-10 = 0.68
          standard error of the difference: 0.05588
          patient stratum concerned: 1

2.  Wide-Excision                      Radical-Mastectomy
    Adjuvant-Radiation-Tx              Adjuvant-Radiation-Tx
    203  patients                      609  patients
    OAS-5 = 0.85                       OAS-5 = 0.8
          standard error of the difference: 0.03744
          patient stratum concerned: 1

3.  Wide-Excision                      Radical-Mastectomy
    Adjuvant-Radiation-Tx              Adjuvant-Radiation-Tx
    203  patients                      609  patients
    RFS-10 = 0.6                       RFS-10 = 0.6
          standard error of the difference: 0.062
          patient stratum concerned: 1

4.  Wide-Excision                      Radical-Mastectomy
    Adjuvant-Radiation-Tx              Adjuvant-Radiation-Tx
    203  patients                      609  patients
    RFS-5 = 0.7                        RFS-5 = 0.7
          standard error of the difference: 0.04659
          patient stratum concerned: 1


The STRATA in peters77:

1.  clinical stages:          (I II)
    tumor sizes:              (TO T1A T1B T2A T2B)
    clinical node staging:    (NO N1A)
    pathologic node staging:  (UNKNOWN)
    metastatic staging:       (MO)
    menopausal status:        (PRE POST)
    age-range:                (20 . 80)


The DISTANCE METRIC KNOWLEDGE in peters77:

    Authors-Conclusions-Incorrect: 1 2 3 4
    Sketchy-Statistical-Reporting: 1 2 3 4
       se-change: INCREASE-SMALL
    Selection-Bias: 1 2 3 4
       se-change: INCREASE-SMALL
    Parallel-Non-Randomized-Controls: 1 2 3 4
       se-change: INCREASE-MODERATE
    Long-Accrual-Period: 1 2 3 4
       se-change: INCREASE-SMALL
```

```
Nonstandard-Intervention: 1 2 3 4
   se-change: NEGLIGIBLE
distance-estimator #7: 1 2 3 4
   dp-change: NEGLIGIBLE
distance-estimator #2: 1 2 3 4
   dp-change: TOWARD-ZERO-SMALL
distance-estimator #1: 1 2 3 4
   dp-change: AWAY-FROM-ZERO-MODERATE
```

Fisher80

```
Reference: [Fisher 80]
Institution: 34 institutions in the U.S. and Canada

The COMPARISONS in Fisher80:

4.  Total-Mastectomy                  Total-Mastectomy
    Adjuvant-Radiation-Tx
    352  patients                     365  patients
    RFS-5 = 0.74                      RFS-5 = 0.66
          standard error of the difference: 0.03727
          patient stratum concerned: 1

5.  Total-Mastectomy                  Total-Mastectomy
    Adjuvant-Radiation-Tx
    352  patients                     365  patients
    OAS-5 = 0.75                      OAS-5 = 0.74
          standard error of the difference: 0.03559
          patient stratum concerned: 1

6.  Radical-Mastectomy                Total-Mastectomy
                                      Adjuvant-Radiation-Tx
    362  patients                     352  patients
    RFS-5 = 0.72                      RFS-5 = 0.74
          standard error of the difference: 0.03624
          patient stratum concerned: 1

7.  Radical-Mastectomy                Total-Mastectomy
                                      Adjuvant-Radiation-Tx
    362  patients                     352  patients
    OAS-5 = 0.75                      OAS-5 = 0.75
          standard error of the difference: 0.03536
          patient stratum concerned: 1

8.  Radical-Mastectomy                Total-Mastectomy
    362  patients                     365  patients
    RFS-5 = 0.72                      RFS-5 = 0.66
          standard error of the difference: 0.03768
          patient stratum concerned: 1

9.  Radical-Mastectomy                Total-Mastectomy
    362  patients                     365  patients
    OAS-5 = 0.75                      OAS-5 = 0.74
          standard error of the difference: 0.03559
          patient stratum concerned: 1
```

```
11. Radical-Mastectomy                   Total-Mastectomy
                                         Adjuvant-Radiation-Tx
    292  patients                        294  patients
    RFS-5 = 0.43                         RFS-5 = 0.48
          standard error of the difference: 0.04448
          patient stratum concerned: 2

12. Radical-Mastectomy                   Total-Mastectomy
                                         Adjuvant-Radiation-Tx
    292  patients                        294  patients
    OAS-5 = 0.62                         OAS-5 = 0.56
          standard error of the difference: 0.04391
          patient stratum concerned: 2


The STRATA in Fisher80:

1.  clinical stages:            (I II III)
    tumor sizes:                (T1A T2A T3A)
    clinical node staging:      (N0 N1A)
    pathologic node staging:    (UNKNOWN)
    metastatic staging:         (M0)
    menopausal status:          (PRE POST)
    age-range:                  (20 . 80)

2.  clinical stages:            (I II III)
    tumor sizes:                (T1A T2A T3A)
    clinical node staging:      (N1B)
    pathologic node staging:    (UNKNOWN)
    metastatic staging:         (M0)
    menopausal status:          (PRE POST)
    age-range:                  (20 . 80)


The DISTANCE METRIC KNOWLEDGE in Fisher80:

    Parallel-Randomized-Controls: 4 5 6 7 8 9 11 12
       se-change: DECREASE-SMALL
    Sketchy-Statistical-Reporting: 4 5 6 7 8 9 11 12
       se-change: NEGLIGIBLE
    Highly-Reliable-Author: 4 5 6 7 8 9 11 12
       se-change: DECREASE-MODERATE
    Modification-Of-Intervention: 4 5 8 9
       se-change: NEGLIGIBLE
    distance-estimator #11: 4 5 6 7 8 9
       se-change: NONE
    distance-estimator #10: 4 5 6 7 8 9
       dp-change: NONE
    distance-estimator #9: 4 5 6 7 8 9
       dp-change: AWAY-FROM-ZERO-MODERATE
    distance-estimator #14: 11 12
       dp-change: TOWARD-ZERO-MODERATE
    distance-estimator #13: 11 12
       dp-change: AWAY-FROM-ZERO-MODERATE
    distance-estimator #12: 11 12
       dp-change: NONE
```

Hellman80

```
Reference: [Hellman 80]
Institution: Joint Center for Radiation Therapy, Boston

The COMPARISONS in Hellman80 :

1.  Wide-Excision                       Intervention-External-To-Study
    Adjuvant-Radiation-Tx
    62  patients                        NIL
    OAS-5 = 0.96                        NIL
          standard error of the difference: 0
          patient stratum concerned: 1

2.  Wide-Excision                       Intervention-External-To-Study
    Adjuvant-Radiation-Tx
    122  patients                       NIL
    OAS-5 = 0.75                        NIL
          standard error of the difference: 0
          patient stratum concerned: 2


The STRATA in Hellman80 :

1.  clinical stages:            (I)
    tumor sizes:                (T0 T1A T1B)
    clinical node staging:      (N0 N1A)
    pathologic node staging:    (UNKNOWN)
    metastatic staging:         (M0)
    menopausal status:          (PRE POST)
    age-range:                  (32 . 81)

2.  clinical stages:            (II)
    tumor sizes:                (T2A T2B)
    clinical node staging:      (N1B)
    pathologic node staging:    (UNKNOWN)
    metastatic staging:         (M0)
    menopausal status:          (PRE POST)
    age-range:                  (32 . 81)


The DISTANCE METRIC KNOWLEDGE in Hellman80 :

    Sketchy-Statistical-Reporting: 1 2
       se-change: INCREASE-SMALL
    Selection-Bias: 1 2
       se-change: INCREASE-MODERATE
    External-Controls: 1 2
       se-change: INCREASE-EXTREME
    Immature-Results: 1
       se-change: INCREASE-MODERATE
    Nonstandard-Outcome: 1 2
       se-change: INCREASE-MODERATE
    Immature-Results: 2
       se-change: INCREASE-MODERATE
    Nonstandard-Intervention: 1
       se-change: INCREASE-SMALL
    Nonstandard-Intervention: 2
```

```
   se-change: INCREASE-SMALL
distance-estimator #5: 1
   se-change: NONE
distance-estimator #4: 2
   se-change: NONE
```

Veronesi81

```
Reference: [Veronesi 81]
Institution: the Cancer Institute in Milan

The COMPARISONS in veronesi81:

1.  Radical-Mastectomy                  We-With-Axillary-Dissection
    Adjuvant-Chemo-If-Histo-Pos         Adjuvant-Radiation-Tx
                                        Adjuvant-Chemo-If-Histo-Pos
    349  patients                       352  patients
    RFS-5 = 0.83                        RFS-5 = 0.84
          standard error of the difference: 0.0396
          patient stratum concerned: 1

2.  Radical-Mastectomy                  We-With-Axillary-Dissection
    Adjuvant-Chemo-If-Histo-Pos         Adjuvant-Radiation-Tx
                                        Adjuvant-Chemo-If-Histo-Pos
    349  patients                       352  patients
    OAS-5 = 0.9                         OAS-5 = 0.9
          standard error of the difference: 0.03607
          patient stratum concerned: 1


The STRATA in veronesi81:

1.  clinical stages:            (I)
    tumor sizes:                (T1A T1B)
    clinical node staging:      (N0)
    pathologic node staging:    (UNKNOWN)
    metastatic staging:         (M0)
    menopausal status:          (PRE POST)
    age-range:                  (20 . 70)


The DISTANCE METRIC KNOWLEDGE in veronesi81:

    Parallel-Randomized-Controls: 1 2
       se-change: DECREASE-SMALL
    distance-estimator #17: 1 2
       dp-change: AWAY-FROM-ZERO-SMALL
    distance-estimator #16: 1 2
       se-change: INCREASE-SMALL
    distance-estimator #15: 1 2
       se-change: NONE
    Nonstandard-Intervention: 1 2
       se-change: NEGLIGIBLE
    distance-estimator #6: 1 2
       dp-change: AWAY-FROM-ZERO-MODERATE
    distance-estimator #5: 1 2
```

```
        se-change: NONE
```

Amalric82

```
Reference: [Amalric 82]
Institution: the Marseilles Cancer Institute

The COMPARISONS in Amalric82:

1.  Wide-Excision                     Radical-Mastectomy
    Adjuvant-Radiation-Tx
    1083 patients                     121  patients
    OAS-5 = 0.73                      OAS-5 = 0.78
          standard error of the difference: 0.04
          patient stratum concerned: 1

2.  Wide-Excision                     Radical-Mastectomy
    Adjuvant-Radiation-Tx
    234  patients                     66   patients
    OAS-10 = 0.68                     OAS-10 = 0.68
          standard error of the difference: 0.06501
          patient stratum concerned: 1


The STRATA in Amalric82:

1.  clinical stages:          (I II)
    tumor sizes:              (UNKNOWN)
    clinical node staging:    (UNKNOWN)
    pathologic node staging:  (UNKNOWN)
    metastatic staging:       (MO)
    menopausal status:        (PRE POST)
    age-range:                (22 . 78)


The DISTANCE METRIC KNOWLEDGE in Amalric82:

    Wide-Stratum: 1 2
       se-change: INCREASE-MODERATE
    Temporal-Drift: 1 2
       se-change: INCREASE-MODERATE
    Parallel-Non-Randomized-Controls: 1 2
       se-change: INCREASE-MODERATE
       dp-change: NEGATIVE-SMALL
    distance-estimator #19: 1 2
       dp-change: AWAY-FROM-ZERO-SMALL
    distance-estimator #18: 1 2
       dp-change: TOWARD-ZERO-SMALL
```

Tapley82

```
Reference: [Tapley 82]
Institution: MD Anderson Hospital

The COMPARISONS in Tapley82:
```

```
1.  Tm-With-Axillary-Dissection        Intervention-External-To-Study
    Adjuvant-Radiation-Tx
    392  patients                      NIL
    RFS-10 = 0.42                      NIL
          standard error of the difference: 0
          patient stratum concerned: 1
```

The STRATA in Tapley82:

```
1.  clinical stages:            (I II)
    tumor sizes:                (UNKNOWN)
    clinical node staging:      (UNKNOWN)
    pathologic node staging:    (0)
    metastatic staging:         (M0)
    menopausal status:          (PRE POST)
    age-range:                  (20 . 80)
```

The DISTANCE METRIC KNOWLEDGE in Tapley82:

```
    Authors-Conclusions-Strong: 1
    External-Controls: 1
       se-change: INCREASE-MODERATE
    Unreliable-Author: 1
       se-change: INCREASE-MODERATE
    Nonstandard-Intervention: 1
       se-change: NEGLIGIBLE
```

Hayward83

Reference: [Hayward 83]
Institution: Guy's Hospital, England

The COMPARISONS in hayward83:

```
1.  Wide-Excision                      Radical-Mastectomy
    Adjuvant-Radiation-Tx              Adjuvant-Radiation-Tx
    121  patients                      132  patients
    LRRF-5 = 0.75                      LRRF-5 = 0.93
          standard error of the difference: 0.0452
          patient stratum concerned: 1

2.  Wide-Excision                      Radical-Mastectomy
    Adjuvant-Radiation-Tx              Adjuvant-Radiation-Tx
    121  patients                      132  patients
    OAS-5 = 0.72                       OAS-5 = 0.85
          standard error of the difference: 0.0513
          patient stratum concerned: 1
```

The STRATA in hayward83:

```
1.  clinical stages:            (I)
    tumor sizes:                (T0 T1A T1B)
```

```
clinical node staging:     (N0 N1A)
pathologic node staging:   (UNKNOWN)
metastatic staging:        (M0)
menopausal status:         (POST)
age-range:                 (50 . 80)
```

The DISTANCE METRIC KNOWLEDGE in hayward83:

```
Parallel-Randomized-Controls: 1 2
   se-change: DECREASE-SMALL
distance-estimator #
   dp-change: NEGATIVE-MODERATE
distance-estimator #6: 1 2
   dp-change: AWAY-FROM-ZERO-MODERATE
distance-estimator #5: 1 2
   se-change: NONE
distance-estimator #3: 1 2
   dp-change: NEGLIGIBLE
```

Fisher85a

Reference: [Fisher 85a]
Institution: multiple NSABP centers

The COMPARISONS in fisher85a:

```
1.  Tm-With-Axillary-Dissection       We-With-Axillary-Dissection
    362  patients                     390  patients
    RFS-5 = 0.72                      RFS-5 = 0.68
           standard error of the difference: 0.0495
           patient stratum concerned: 1

2.  Tm-With-Axillary-Dissection       We-With-Axillary-Dissection
    362  patients                     390  patients
    OAS-5 = 0.82                      OAS-5 = 0.91
           standard error of the difference: 0.04579
           patient stratum concerned: 1

3.  Tm-With-Axillary-Dissection       We-With-Axillary-Dissection
                                      Adjuvant-Radiation-Tx
    362  patients                     396  patients
    RFS-5 = 0.72                      RFS-5 = 0.81
           standard error of the difference: 0.04545
           patient stratum concerned: 1

4.  Tm-With-Axillary-Dissection       We-With-Axillary-Dissection
                                      Adjuvant-Radiation-Tx
    362  patients                     396  patients
    OAS-5 = 0.82                      OAS-5 = 0.92
           standard error of the difference: 0.04429
           patient stratum concerned: 1

5.  We-With-Axillary-Dissection       We-With-Axillary-Dissection
                                      Adjuvant-Radiation-Tx
    358  patients                     373  patients
```

```
    RFS-5 = 0.68                        RFS-5 = 0.81
           standard error of the difference: 0.04763
           patient stratum concerned: 3

6.  We-With-Axillary-Dissection         We-With-Axillary-Dissection
                                        Adjuvant-Radiation-Tx
    358  patients                       373  patients
    OAS-5 = 0.9                         OAS-5 = 0.91
           standard error of the difference: 0.0333
           patient stratum concerned: 3

7.  We-With-Axillary-Dissection         We-With-Axillary-Dissection
                                        Adjuvant-Radiation-Tx
    358  patients                       373  patients
    IPSI-RFS-5 = 0.77                   IPSI-RFS-5 = 0.9
           standard error of the difference: 0.03982
           patient stratum concerned: 3

8.  Tm-With-Axillary-Dissection         We-With-Axillary-Dissection
    Adjuvant-Chemo                      Adjuvant-Chemo
    224  patients                       242  patients
    RFS-5 = 0.58                        RFS-5 = 0.55
           standard error of the difference: 0.07783
           patient stratum concerned: 2

9.  Tm-With-Axillary-Dissection         We-With-Axillary-Dissection
    Adjuvant-Chemo                      Adjuvant-Chemo
    224  patients                       242  patients
    OAS-5 = 0.66                        OAS-5 = 0.74
           standard error of the difference: 0.07495
           patient stratum concerned: 2

10. Tm-With-Axillary-Dissection         We-With-Axillary-Dissection
    Adjuvant-Chemo                      Adjuvant-Radiation-Tx
                                        Adjuvant-Chemo
    224  patients                       229  patients
    RFS-5 = 0.58                        RFS-5 = 0.58
           standard error of the difference: 0.07566
           patient stratum concerned: 2

11. Tm-With-Axillary-Dissection         We-With-Axillary-Dissection
    Adjuvant-Chemo                      Adjuvant-Radiation-Tx
                                        Adjuvant-Chemo
    224  patients                       229  patients
    OAS-5 = 0.66                        OAS-5 = 0.75
           standard error of the difference: 0.06953
           patient stratum concerned: 2

12. We-With-Axillary-Dissection         We-With-Axillary-Dissection
    Adjuvant-Chemo                      Adjuvant-Radiation-Tx
                                        Adjuvant-Chemo
    207  patients                       193  patients
    RFS-5 = 0.57                        RFS-5 = 0.61
           standard error of the difference: 0.08345
           patient stratum concerned: 4

13. We-With-Axillary-Dissection         We-With-Axillary-Dissection
    Adjuvant-Chemo                      Adjuvant-Radiation-Tx
```

```
                                         Adjuvant-Chemo
    207  patients                        193  patients
    OAS-5 = 0.74                         OAS-5 = 0.79
           standard error of the difference: 0.07106
           patient stratum concerned: 4

14. We-With-Axillary-Dissection          We-With-Axillary-Dissection
    Adjuvant-Chemo                       Adjuvant-Radiation-Tx
                                         Adjuvant-Chemo
    207  patients                        193  patients
    IPSI-RFS-5 = 0.64                    IPSI-RFS-5 = 0.98
           standard error of the difference: 0.0592
           patient stratum concerned: 4


The STRATA in fisher85a:

1.  clinical stages:             (I II)
    tumor sizes:                 (TO T1A T2A)
    clinical node staging:       (NO N1A N1B)
    pathologic node staging:     (0)
    metastatic staging:          (MO)
    menopausal status:           (PRE POST)
    age-range:                   (20 . 80)

2.  clinical stages:             (I II)
    tumor sizes:                 (TO T1A T2A)
    clinical node staging:       (NO N1A N1B)
    pathologic node staging:     (1 2 3 4UP)
    metastatic staging:          (MO)
    menopausal status:           (PRE POST)
    age-range:                   (20 . 80)

3.  clinical stages:             (I II)
    tumor sizes:                 (TO T1A T2A)
    clinical node staging:       (NO N1A N1B)
    pathologic node staging:     (0)
    metastatic staging:          (MO)
    menopausal status:           (PRE POST)
    age-range:                   (20 . 80)

4.  clinical stages:             (I II)
    tumor sizes:                 (TO T1A T2A)
    clinical node staging:       (NO N1A N1B)
    pathologic node staging:     (1 2 3 4UP)
    metastatic staging:          (MO)
    menopausal status:           (PRE POST)
    age-range:                   (20 . 80)


The DISTANCE METRIC KNOWLEDGE in fisher85a:

    Parallel-Randomized-Controls: 1 2 3 4 5 6 7 8 9 10 11 12
13 14
       se-change: DECREASE-SMALL
    Highly-Reliable-Author: 1 2 3 4 5 6 7 8 9 10 11 12 13 14
       se-change: DECREASE-SMALL
    Nonstandard-Outcome: 1 3 5 8 10 12
```

```
   dp-change: TOWARD-ZERO-MODERATE
Authors-Conclusions-Strong: 3 4 10 11
distance-estimator #17: 1 2 3 4 5 6 7 8 9 10 11 12 13 14
   dp-change: AWAY-FROM-ZERO-SMALL
distance-estimator #16: 1 2 3 4 5 6 7 8 9 10 11 12 13 14
   se-change: INCREASE-SMALL
distance-estimator #15: 1 2 3 4 5 6 7 8 9 10 11 12 13 14
   se-change: NONE
Modification-Of-Intervention: 1 2 3 4 8 9 10 11
   se-change: INCREASE-MODERATE
Nonstandard-Intervention: 3 4 5 6 7 10 11 12 13 14
   se-change: NEGLIGIBLE
distance-estimator #20: 1 2 3 4 5 6 7
   dp-change: TOWARD-ZERO-MODERATE
distance-estimator #23: 5 6 7 12 13 14
   se-change: DECREASE-SMALL
   dp-change: NONE
distance-estimator #22: 5 6 7 12 13 14
   dp-change: AWAY-FROM-ZERO-MODERATE
distance-estimator #21: 8 9 10 11 12 13 14
   dp-change: AWAY-FROM-ZERO-MODERATE
```

Fisher85b

```
Reference: [Fisher 85b]
Institution: 34 institutions in the U.S. and Canada

The COMPARISONS in Fisher85b:

1.  Total-Mastectomy                 Total-Mastectomy
    Adjuvant-Radiation-Tx
    352  patients                    365  patients
    LRRF-10 = 0.95                   LRRF-10 = 0.85
          standard error of the difference: 0.02201
          patient stratum concerned: 1

2.  Radical-Mastectomy               Total-Mastectomy
                                     Adjuvant-Radiation-Tx
    362  patients                    352  patients
    LRRF-10 = 0.9                    LRRF-10 = 0.95
          standard error of the difference: 0.01958
          patient stratum concerned: 1

3.  Radical-Mastectomy               Total-Mastectomy
    362  patients                    365  patients
    LRRF-10 = 0.9                    LRRF-10 = 0.85
          standard error of the difference: 0.02445
          patient stratum concerned: 1

4.  Total-Mastectomy                 Total-Mastectomy
    Adjuvant-Radiation-Tx
    352  patients                    365  patients
    RFS-10 = 0.48                    RFS-10 = 0.42
          standard error of the difference: 0.03748
          patient stratum concerned: 1
```

```
5.  Total-Mastectomy                     Total-Mastectomy
    Adjuvant-Radiation-Tx
    352  patients                        365  patients
    OAS-10 = 0.59                        OAS-10 = 0.54
          standard error of the difference: 0.03818
          patient stratum concerned: 1

6.  Radical-Mastectomy                   Total-Mastectomy
                                         Adjuvant-Radiation-Tx
    362  patients                        352  patients
    RFS-10 = 0.47                        RFS-10 = 0.48
          standard error of the difference: 0.03748
          patient stratum concerned: 1

7.  Radical-Mastectomy                   Total-Mastectomy
                                         Adjuvant-Radiation-Tx
    362  patients                        352  patients
    OAS-10 = 0.58                        OAS-10 = 0.59
          standard error of the difference: 0.03748
          patient stratum concerned: 1

8.  Radical-Mastectomy                   Total-Mastectomy
    362  patients                        365  patients
    RFS-10 = 0.47                        RFS-10 = 0.42
          standard error of the difference: 0.03677
          patient stratum concerned: 1

9.  Radical-Mastectomy                   Total-Mastectomy
    362  patients                        365  patients
    OAS-10 = 0.58                        OAS-10 = 0.54
          standard error of the difference: 0.03748
          patient stratum concerned: 1

10. Radical-Mastectomy                   Total-Mastectomy
                                         Adjuvant-Radiation-Tx
    292  patients                        294  patients
    LRRF-10 = 0.85                       LRRF-10 = 0.86
          standard error of the difference: 0.02909
          patient stratum concerned: 2

11. Radical-Mastectomy                   Total-Mastectomy
                                         Adjuvant-Radiation-Tx
    292  patients                        294  patients
    RFS-10 = 0.29                        RFS-10 = 0.25
          standard error of the difference: 0.03748
          patient stratum concerned: 2

12. Radical-Mastectomy                   Total-Mastectomy
                                         Adjuvant-Radiation-Tx
    292  patients                        294  patients
    OAS-10 = 0.38                        OAS-10 = 0.39
          standard error of the difference: 0.04101
          patient stratum concerned: 2


The STRATA in Fisher85b:

1.  clinical stages:          (I II III)
```

```
    tumor sizes:               (T1A T2A T3A)
    clinical node staging:     (NO N1A)
    pathologic node staging:   (UNKNOWN)
    metastatic staging:        (MO)
    menopausal status:         (PRE POST)
    age-range:                 (20 . 80)

2.  clinical stages:           (I II III)
    tumor sizes:               (T1A T2A T3A)
    clinical node staging:     (N1B)
    pathologic node staging:   (UNKNOWN)
    metastatic staging:        (MO)
    menopausal status:         (PRE POST)
    age-range:                 (20 . 80)


The DISTANCE METRIC KNOWLEDGE in Fisher85b:

    Parallel-Randomized-Controls: 1 2 3 4 5 6 7 8 9 10 11 12
       se-change: DECREASE-SMALL
    Sketchy-Statistical-Reporting: 1 2 3 10
       se-change: INCREASE-MODERATE
    Highly-Reliable-Author: 1 2 3 4 5 6 7 8 9 10 11 12
       se-change: DECREASE-MODERATE
    Modification-Of-Intervention: 1 3 4 5 8 9
       se-change: NEGLIGIBLE
    distance-estimator #11: 1 2 3 4 5 6 7 8 9
       se-change: NONE
    distance-estimator #10: 1 2 3 4 5 6 7 8 9
       dp-change: NONE
    distance-estimator #9: 1 2 3 4 5 6 7 8 9
       dp-change: AWAY-FROM-ZERO-MODERATE
    distance-estimator #14: 10 11 12
       dp-change: TOWARD-ZERO-MODERATE
    distance-estimator #13: 10 11 12
       dp-change: AWAY-FROM-ZERO-MODERATE
    distance-estimator #12: 10 11 12
       dp-change: NONE
```

Appendix II
Sample Distance Estimators

This appendix shows several example distance estimators from the Roundsman system. There are two types of distance estimators: *population* distance estimators are used to assess population mismatches while *intervention* distance estimators are used to assess intervention mismatches. (Population mismatches and intervention mismatches are discussed more fully in section 4.2.)

The example distance estimators in this appendix are shown in the following format:

```
(a  TYPE OF DISTANCE ESTIMATOR  with
     slotname  =  (SLOTVALUEs)
     slotname  =  (SLOTVALUEs)
       ...
  )
```

The slot values are *equivalence classes* which are defined on outcomes, interventions, population descriptions and patient descriptions. The slot *values* allow the distance estimator to determine whether it can contribute to the distance assessment between a particular *comparison* (see appendix I for examples of comparison objects) and the physician's patient and treatment plan.

The use of equivalence classes allows the distance estimators to apply to *sets* of outcomes, *sets* of interventions, etc. The equivalence class approach also allows the Roundsman system to adapt flexibly to changes that occur over time, for example the addition of a new intervention object when a newly-encoded clinical study uses an intervention that has not previously been part of the knowledge base. Roundsman's equivalence class definitions are updated in order to define to which class(es) the new intervention belongs. The pre-existing distance estimators can then continue to operate without interruption. Slot values do not have to be examined individually and altered to accommodate the new intervention.

[*In this appendix, explanatory text is italicized and enclosed in brackets.*]

```
(a  POPULATION-DISTANCE-ESTIMATOR  with
   outcome-eq-classes           = (OAS)
   intervention1-eq-classes     = (ANY)
   intervention2-eq-classes     = (ANY)
   study-pop-classes            = (T1-2  NO-1A)
   patient-classes              = (CLINICAL-STAGE-I)
   bias-incurred   =
```

```
(a WORSE-PROGNOSTIC-STRATUM  with
  dp-change = TOWARD-ZERO-SMALL
  specifics =
  "this group had negative clinical node exams like
   your patient, but was composed of BOTH T1 and T2"
   ))
```

[*The distance estimator shown above evaluates whether the outcome under consideration is a member of the OAS (overall survival) equivalence class. Examples of outcomes which belong to the OAS class are overall survival at five years and overall survival at ten years. The next two slots specify the intervention equivalence class ANY, which means that this distance estimator applies to any interventions in the Roundsman system. The values of the "study-pop-classes" slot specify that the study population must be a group that includes both T1 and T2 tumor sizes (equivalence class T1-2) and also includes both N0 and N1a axillary node statuses (equivalence class N0-1A). Finally, the patient being considered must be clinical stage I by clinical exam (equivalence class CLINICAL-STAGE-I).*]

[*If these equivalence class membership conditions are met, then this distance estimator augments the distance metric of the comparison object with a population mismatch of type "worse-prognostic-stratum". (Distance metric components are discussed more fully in sections 4.2 and 4.3.) When all applicable distance estimators have built up the distance metric in this manner, Roundsman uses the components collected in the distance metric to assess the relevance of the statistical results to the physician's clinical problem (treatment plan and patient).*]

```
(an  INTERVENTION-DISTANCE-ESTIMATOR  with
   outcome-eq-classes              =  (OAS)
   population-eq-classes           =  (ANY)
   studied-intervention-classes    =  (CHEMO-IF-POS)
   proposed-intervention-classes =  (NOCHEMO)
   bias-incurred  =
      (an ADDITION-OF-BENEFICIAL-MODALITY  with
       dp-change =  AWAY-FROM-ZERO-SMALL
       specifics =
        "chemotherapy was given if axillary nodes were histo+"
        ))
```

[*The distance estimator shown above is activated if the outcome belongs to the OAS equivalence class, if the study intervention belongs to the CHEMO-IF-POS equivalence class and the physician's plan belongs to the NOCHEMO equivalence class. Upon activation, this distance estimator augments the distance metric of the comparison object with an intervention mismatch of type "addition-of-beneficial-modality" with slot values as shown.*]

```
(an  INTERVENTION-DISTANCE-ESTIMATOR  with
     outcome-eq-classes               =  (OAS)
     population-eq-classes            =  (ANY)
     studied-intervention-classes     =  (CHEMO-IF-POS)
     proposed-intervention-classes =     (CHEMO-IF-POS)
     bias-incurred  =
       (a SAME-ADJUVANT-MODALITY-USED  with
          se-change = NONE
          specifics =
           "chemotherapy given if axillary nodes are path. positive"
       ))


(a  POPULATION-DISTANCE-ESTIMATOR  with
    outcome-eq-classes           = (OAS)
    intervention1-eq-classes     = (ANY)
    intervention2-eq-classes     = (ANY)
    study-pop-classes            = (CLINICAL-STAGES-I-II )
    patient-classes              = (CLINICAL-STAGE-II )
    bias-incurred   =
       (a  BETTER-PROGNOSTIC-STRATUM
         dp-change = AWAY-FROM-ZERO-SMALL
         specifics =
         "the study used a pooled clinical stage I and II -  so that's
           a slightly better prognostic group than your patient"
         ))


(a  POPULATION-DISTANCE-ESTIMATOR  with
    outcome-eq-classes           = (OAS)
    intervention1-eq-classes     = (ANY)
    intervention2-eq-classes     = (ANY)
    study-pop-classes            = (PATH-NODE-NEG)
    patient-classes              = (CLINICAL-STAGE-I)
    bias-incurred   =
       (a  BETTER-PROGNOSTIC-STRATUM
         dp-change = AWAY-FROM-ZERO-MODERATE
         specifics =
         "this study stratum was defined by negative axillary node
           histology; about 40% of  clinical stage I patients like
           yours will have positive histology"
         ))


(a  POPULATION-DISTANCE-ESTIMATOR  with
    outcome-eq-classes           = (ANY)
    intervention1-eq-classes     = (ANY)
    intervention2-eq-classes     = (ANY)
    study-pop-classes            = (VERIFIED-WIDE-EXCISION)
    patient-classes              = (NOT-VERIFIED-WIDE-EXCISION)
```

```
    bias-incurred   =
       (a WORSE-PROGNOSTIC-STRATUM
         dp-change = TOWARD-ZERO-MODERATE
         specifics =
         "if a woman's excision margins contained any tumor
          (by path exam), she was excluded from this group"
         ))


(an  INTERVENTION-DISTANCE-ESTIMATOR  with
     outcome-eq-classes               = (OAS)
     population-eq-classes            = (ANY)
     studied-intervention-classes     = (ADJ-RTX)
     proposed-intervention-classes    = (NO-ADJ-RTX)
     bias-incurred  =
        (an ADDITION-OF-BENEFICIAL-MODALITY
         se-change = INCREASE-EXTREME
         specifics =
          "unless you use adjuvant radiotherapy as they did
           in this study, it is questionable whether these
           results can be used for your case"
       ))


(a  POPULATION-DISTANCE-ESTIMATOR  with
    outcome-eq-classes          = (OAS)
    intervention1-eq-classes    = (ANY)
    intervention2-eq-classes    = (ANY)
    study-pop-classes           = (CLINICAL-STAGE-I)
    patient-classes             = (CLINICAL-STAGE-II)
    bias-incurred   =
       (a BETTER-PROGNOSTIC-STRATUM with
         specifics = "they were clinically stage I"
         dp-change = 'AWAY-FROM-ZERO-MODERATE )
         ))


  (a  POPULATION-DISTANCE-ESTIMATOR  with
      outcome-eq-classes          = (OAS)
      intervention1-eq-classes    = (ANY)
      intervention2-eq-classes    = (ANY)
      study-pop-classes           = (T1-2-3  N1b)
      patient-classes             = (CLINICAL-STAGE-I)
      bias-incurred   =
         (a WORSE-PROGNOSTIC-STRATUM
          dp-change = TOWARD-ZERO-MODERATE
          specifics =
          "they included T1, T2 or T3 and they were all
           clinically node positive"
         ))
```

```
(an  INTERVENTION-DISTANCE-ESTIMATOR  with
     outcome-eq-classes              =  (OAS)
     population-eq-classes           =  (ANY)
     studied-intervention-classes    =  (CHEMO-IF-POS)
     proposed-intervention-classes   =  (CHEMO)
     bias-incurred  =
        (a  MODALITY-SLIGHTLY-DISSIMILAR   with
         se-change = INCREASE-SMALL
         specifics =
         "patients in this study received chemo ONLY if axillary nodes
          were histologically positive")
       ))
```

REFERENCES

[Aikins 83] Aikins, J. S., Kunz, J.C., Shortliffe, E.H. and Fallat, R. J.
An expert system for interpretation of pulmonary function data.
Computers and Biomedical Research 16:199-208, 1983.

[Albert 81] Albert, D. A.
Deciding whether the conclusions of studies are justified: a review.
Medical Decision Making 1(3):265-275, 1981.

[Amalric 82] Amalric, R., et al.
Radiation therapy with or without primary limited surgery for operable breast cancer: A 20-year experience at the Marseilles Cancer Institute.
Cancer 49:30-34, 1982.

[Atkins 72] Atkins, H. , Hayward, J. L., et al.
Treatment of early breast cancer: a report after ten years of a clinical trial.
British Medical Journal 2:423-429, 1972.

[Bailar 84a] Bailar, J. C., Louis, T. A., Lavori, P. W. and Polansky, M.
Studies without internal controls.
New England Journal of Medicine 311:156-62, 1984.

[Bailar 84b] Bailar, J. C., Louis, T. A., Lavori, P. W. and Polansky, M.
A classification for biomedical research reports.
New England Journal of Medicine 311:1482-7, 1984.

[Bailar 85] Bailar, J. C.
When research results are in conflict.
New England Journal of Medicine 313:1080-1081, 1985.

[Barnett 84] Barnett, G. O.
The application of computer-based medical-record systems in ambulatory practice.
New England Journal of Medicine 310:1643-1650, 1984.

[Beck 82] Beck, J. R., Kassirer, J. P. and Pauker, S. G.
A convenient approximation of life expectancy (The 'DEALE').
American Journal of Medicine 73:883-97, 1982.

[Begg 85] Begg, C. B.
A measure to aid in the interpretation of published clinical studies.
Statistics in Medicine 4(1):1-9, 1985.

[Bernstein 80] Bernstein, L. M., Seigel, E. R., and Goldstein, C. M.
The hepatitis knowledge base: a prototype information transfer system.
Annals of Internal Medicine 93(2):169-181, 1980.

[Blum 82] Blum, R. L.
Discovery, confirmation, and incorporation of causal relationships from a large time-oriented clincal data base: the RX project.
Computers and Biomedical Research 15:164-187, 1982.
also published in [Clancey 84a].

[Brinkley 66] Brinkley, D. and Haybittle, J. L.
Treatment of stage-II carcinoma of the female breast.
Lancet 2:291-295, 1966.

[Brinkley 71] Brinkley, D. and Haybittle, J. L.
Treatment of stage-II carcinoma of the female breast.
Lancet 2:1086-1087, 1971.

[Brown 82] Brown, J.S., Burton, R.R. and de Kleer, J.
Pedagogical, natural language, and knowledge engineering techniques in SOPHIE I, II, and III.
Academic Press, London, 1982, pages 227-282, .

[Buchanan 78] Buchanan, B. G. and Feigenbaum, E. A.
DENDRAL and Meta-DENDRAL: their applications dimension.
Artificial Intelligence 11(1):5-24, 1978.

[Buchanan 84] Buchanan, B. G. and Shortliffe, E. H. (editors).
Rule-Based Expert Systems: The MYCIN Experiments of the Stanford Heuristic Programming Project.
Addison-Wesley, Reading, MA, 1984.

[Chalmers 81] Chalmers, T. C, Smith H. Jr., Blackburn, B., Silverman, B., Schroeder, B., Reitman, D. and Ambroz, A.
A method for assessing the quality of a randomized control trial.
Controlled Clinical Trials 2:31-49, 1981.

[Clancey 81] Clancey, W. J. and Letsinger, R.
NEOMYCIN: Reconfiguring a Rule-Based Expert System for Application to Teaching.
In *Proceedings of the Seventh International Joint Conferences on Artificial Intelligence*, pages 829-836. IJCAI, 1981.
(Also appears in [Clancey 84a]).

[Clancey 83] Clancey, W.J.
The epistemology of a rule-based expert system: A framework for explanation.
Artificial Intelligence 20:215-251, 1983.

[Clancey 84a] Clancey, W. J. and Shortliffe, E. H. (editors).
Readings in Medical Artificial Intelligence.
Addison-Wesley Publishing Company, Reading, MA., 1984.

[Clancey 84b] Clancey, W. J.
Classification problem solving.
In *Proceedings of the National Conference on Artificial Intelligence*, pages 49-55. American Association for Artificial Intelligence, 1984.

[Clancey 84c] Clancey, W. J.
Details of the revised therapy algorithm.
In Buchanan and Shortliffe (editors), *Rule-Based Expert Systems*, . Addison-Wesley Publishing Company, Reading, MA, 1984.

[Colton 74] Colton, T.
Statistics in Medicine.
Little, Brown and Company, Boston, 1974.

[Cooper 84] Cooper G. F.
NESTOR: A Computer-Based Medical Diagnostic Aid that Integrates Causal and Probabilistic Knowledge.
PhD thesis, Stanford University, 1984.

[Cox 72] Cox, D. R.
Regression models and life-tables.
Journal of the Royal Statistical Society 34:187-220, 1972.

[Critchfield 86] Critchfield, G. C. and Willard, K. E.
Probabilistic sensitivity analysis of decision trees using Monte Carlo simulation.
Medical Decision Making 6:85-92, 1986.

[Davis 79] Davis, R.
Interactive transfer of expertise: Acquisition of new inference rules.
Artificial Intelligence 12:121-158, 1979.

[Davis 84] Davis, R.
Diagnostic reasoning based on structure and behavior.
Artificial Intelligence 24:347-410, 1984.

[deDombal 86] deDombal, F. T., Clamp, S. E., Softley, A, et al.
Prediction of individual patient prognosis: Value of computer-aided systems.
Medical Decision Making 6:18-22, 1986.

[Doszkocs 80] Doszkocs, T. E., Rapp, B. A. and Schoolman, H. M.
Automated information retrieval in science and technology.
Science 208(4):25-30, 1980.

[Doubilet 83] Doubilet, P., McNeil, B. J. and Weinstein, M. C.
Optimal strategies for the diagnosis and treatment of coronary artery disease: analysis using microcomputer.
Medical Decision Making 3(1):23-28, 1983.

[Doubilet 85] Doubilet, P., Begg, C. B., Weinstein, M. C., et al. .
Probabilistic sensitivity analysis using Monte Carlo simulation: a practical approach.
Medical Decision Making 5:157-177, 1985.

[E. Fisher 86] Fisher, E. R., Sass, R., Fisher, B. et al.
Pathologic findings from the national surgical adjuvant breast project (protocol 6).
Cancer 57:1717-1724, 1986.

[Elstein 78] Elstein, A. S., Shulman, L. S., and Sprafka, S. A.
Medical Problem Solving: An Analysis of Clinical Reasoning.
Harvard University Press, Cambridge, 1978.

[Fagan 79] Fagan, L. M., Kunz, J. C., Feigenbaum, E. A. and Osborn, J. J.
Representation of dynamic clinical knowledge: measurement interpretation in the intensive care unit.
In *Proceedings of the Sixth International Joint Conferences on Artificial Intelligence*, pages 260-262. 1979.
(An edited version appears in [Buchanan 84]).

[Feinstein 83] Feinstein, A. R.
An additional basic science for clinical medicine: I. the constraining fundamental paradigms. II. the limitations of randomized trials. III. the challenges of comparison and measurement. IV. the development of clinimetrics.
Annals of Internal Medicine 99:393-397, 544-550, 705-712, 843-848, 1983.

[Feinstein 85] Feinstein, A. R., Sosin, D., M. and Wells, C. K.
Stage migration and new diagnostic techniques as a source of misleading statistics for survival in cancer.
New England Journal of Medicine 312:1604-8, 1985.

[Feltovich 80] Feltovich, P. J., Johnson, P. E., Moller, J. H., and Swanson, D. B.
The role and development of medical knowledge in diagnostic expertise.
1980.
Paper presented at the 1980 annual meeting of the American Educational Research Association (Also appears in [Clancey 84a]).

[Fisher 70] Fisher, B., Slack, N. H., Cavanaugh, P. J. et al.
Postoperative radiotherapy in the treatment of breast cancer: Results of the NSABP clinical trial.
Annals of Surgery 172:711-730, 1970.

[Fisher 77] Fisher, B., Montague, E., Redmond, C. et al.
Comparison of radical mastectomy with alternative treatments for primary breast cancer: A first report of results from a prospective randomized clinical trial.
Cancer 39:2827-2839, 1977.

[Fisher 80] Fisher, B. Redmond, C., Fisher, E. R. et al. .
The contribution of recent NSABP clincal trials of primary breast cancer to an understanding of tumor biology - an overview of findings.
Cancer 46:1009-1025, 1980.

[Fisher 85a] Fisher, B. , Bauer, M. Margolese, R. et al.
Five-year results of a randomized clinical trial comparing total mastectomy and segmental mastectomy with or without radiation in the treatment of breast cancer.
New England Journal of Medicine 312:665-673, March, 1985.

[Fisher 85b] Fisher, B. Redmond, C., Fisher, E. R. et al. .
Ten-year results of a randomized clinical trial comparing radical mastectomy and total mastectomy with or without radiation.
New England Journal of Medicine 312:674-681, 1985.

[Gale 82] Gale, W. A. and Pregibon, D.
An Expert System for Regression Analysis.
In Heiner, K. W. (editor), *Computer Science and Statistics: Proceedings of 14th Symposium on the Interface*, . Springer-Verlag, New York, 1982.

[Gardner 84] Gardner, A. L.
An Artificial Intelligence Approach to Legal Reasoning.
PhD thesis, Stanford University, 1984.

[Genesereth 84] Genesereth, M. R.
The use of design descriptions in automated diagnosis.
Artificial Intelligence 24:411-436, 1984.

[Gomez 81] Gomez, F. and Chandrasekaran, B.
Knowledge organization and distribution for medical diagnosis.
IEEE Transactions on Systems, Man and Cybernetics SMC-11(1):34-42, 1981.

[Gorry 73] Gorry, G. A., Kassirer, J. P., Essig, A., and Schwartz, W. B.
Decision analysis as the basis for computer-aided management of acute renal failure.
American Journal of Medicine 55:473-484, 1973.

[Gorry 78] Gorry, G. A., Silverman, H., and Pauker, S. G.
Capturing clinical expertise: a computer program that considers clinical responses to digitalis.
American Journal of Medicine 64:452-460, 1978.

[Haagensen 63] Haagensen, C. D. and Cooley, E.
Radical mastectomy for mammary carcinoma.
Annals of Surgery 157:166-169, 1963.

[Haagensen 69] Haagensen, C. D. and Cooley, E.
Radical mastectomy for mammary carcinoma.
Annals of Surgery 170:884-888, 1969.

[Haggarty 84] Haggarty, J.
REFEREE and RULECRITIC: Two prototypes for assessing the quality of a medical paper.
Master's thesis, Stanford University, 1984.

[Hajek 82] Hajek, P. and Ivanek, J.
Artificial intelligence and data analysis.
In *COMPSTAT*, pages 54-60. Physica-Verlag, Vienna for the International Association for Statistical Computing, 1982.

[Halvorsen 83] Halvorsen, K. T.
Estimation of Population Parameters Using Information From Several Independent Sources.
PhD thesis, Harvard School of Public Health, 1983.

[Handley 63] Handley, R. S. and Thackray, A. C.
Conservative radical mastectomy (Patey's operation).
Annals of Surgery 157:162-164, 1963.

[Handley 69] Handley, R. S. and Thackray, A. C.
Conservative radical mastectomy (Patey's operation).
Annals of Surgery 170:880-882, 1969.

[Hasling 84] Hasling, D. W., Clancey, W. J. and Rennels, G. D.
Strategic explanations for a diagnostic consulting system.
International Journal of Man-Machine Studies 20:3-19, 1984.

[Hayes-Roth 83] Hayes-Roth, F, Waterman, D, and Lenat. D (eds).
Building Expert Systems.
Addison-Wesley, Reading, MA, 1983.

[Hayward 77] Hayward, J. L.
The Guy's trial of treatments of 'early' breast cancer.
World Journal of Surgery 1:314-316, 1977.

[Hayward 83] Hayward, J. L.
The Guy's Hospital Trials on Breast Conservation.
In Harris, J. R., Hellman, S. and Silen, W. (editors), *Conservative Management of Breast Cancer*, . J.P. Lippincott Company, Philadelphia, 1983.

[Hellman 80] Hellman, S., Harris, J. R. and Levene, M. B.
Radiation therapy of early carcinoma of the breast without mastectomy.
Cancer 46:988-994, 1980.

[Hickam 85] Hickam, D. H., Shortliffe, E. H., Bischoff, M. B., Scott, A. C. and Jacobs, C. D.
The treatment advice of a computer-based cancer chemotherapy protocol advisor.
Annals of Internal Medicine 103:928-936, 1985.

[Hirschman 81] Hirschman, L., Story, G, Marsh, E. Lyman, M. and Sager, N.
An experiment in automated health care evaluation from narrative medical records.
Computers and Biomedical Research 14(5):447-463, 1981.

[Hollenberg 84] Hollenberg, J. P.
The decision tree builder: An expert system to simulate medical prognosis and management.
Medical Decision Making 4(4):531, 1984.
(Abstract).

[Horowitz 81] Horowitz, G. L. and Bleich, H. L.
Paperchase: a computer program to search the medical literature.
New England Journal of Medicine 305:924-930, 1981.

[Howard 70] Howard, R. A.
Decision analysis: perspectives on inference, decision, and experimentation.
In *Proceedings of the IEEE.* IEEE, May, 1970.

[Hwang 81] Hwang, C. and Kwangsun, Y.
Multiple Attribute Decision Making.
Springer-Verlag, New York, 1981.
Lecture Notes in Economics and Mathematical Systems.

[Ingelfinger 83] Ingelfinger, J. A., Mosteller, F., Thibodeau, L. A. and Ware, J. H.
Biostatistics in Clinical Medicine.
MacMillan Publishing Co., Inc., New York, 1983.

[Kaee 65] Kaee, S. and Johansen, H.
Simple mastectomy plus postoperative irradiation by the method of McWhirter for mammary carcinoma.
In Ariel, I. M. (editor), *Progress in Clinical Cancer*, pages 453-461. Grune & Stratton, New York, 1965.

[Kassirer 78] Kassirer, J. P., and Gorry, G. A.
Clinical problem solving: a behavioral analysis.
Annals of Internal Medicine 89:245-255, 1978.

[Kassirer 82] Kassirer, J.P., Kuipers, B.J. and Gorry, G.A.
Toward a theory of clinical expertise.
American Journal of Medicine 73:251-259, 1982.

[Kastner 81] Kastner, J. K.
A precedence scheme for selection and explanation of therapies.
In *Proceedings of the Seventh International Joint Conferences on Artificial Intelligence*, pages 908-909. IJCAI, 1981.

[Kastner 83] Kastner, J. K.
Strategies for Expert Consultation in Therapy Planning.
PhD thesis, Rutgers University, 1983.
Laboratory for Computer Science Research, CBM-TR-136.

[Keeney 76] Keeney, R. and Raiffa, H.
Decisions with Multiple Objectives: Preferences and Value Trade-offs.
John Wiley & Sons, New York, 1976.

[Kolata 84] Kolata, G.
Does a lack of calcium cause hypertension?
Science 225(4663):705-706, 1984.

[KROC 84] The KROC Collaborative Study Group.
Blood glucose control and the evolution of diabetic retinopathy and albuminuria.
New England Journal of Medicine 311(6):365-372, 1984.

[Kuipers 84] Kuipers, B.J. and Kassirer J.P.
Causal reasoning in medicine: Analysis of a protocol.
Cognitive Science 8:363-385, 1984.

[Kulikowski 82] Kulikowski, C., and Weiss, S.
Representation of expert knowledge for consultation: The CASNET and EXPERT projects.
In P. Szolovits (editor), *Artificial intelligence in medicine*, pages 21-55. Westview Press, Boulder, Colo., 1982.

[Lavori 83] Lavori, P. W., Louis, T. A., Bailar, J. C. III and Polansky, M.
Design for experiments - parallel comparisons of treatment.
New England Journal of Medicine 309(21):1291-1298, 1983.

[Ledley 59] Ledley, R. S. and Lusted, L. B.
Reasoning foundations of medical diagnosis.
Science 130:9-21, 1959.

[Levene 77] Levene, M. B., Harris, J. R. and Hellman, S.
Treatment of carcinoma of the breast by radiation therapy.
Cancer 39:2840-2845, 1977.

[Lindgren 76] Lindgren, B. W.
Statistical Theory.
Macmillan Publishing Co., Inc., New York, 1976.
third edition.

[Long 84] Long, W. J., Naimi, S., Criscitiello, M. G., Pauker, S. G. and Szolovits, P.
An aid to physiological reasoning in the management of cardiovascular disease.
In *Proceedings of the IEEE Computers in Cardiology Conference*, pages 3-6. IEEE, 1984.

[McCarron 84] McCarron, D. A., Morris, C. D., Henry, H. J. and Stanton, J. L.
Blood pressure and nutrient intake in the United States.
Science 224(4656):1392-1398, 1984.

[McKeown 85] McKeown, K. R.
Discourse strategies for generating natural-language text.
Artificial Intelligence 27:1-41, 1985.

[McNeil 75] McNeil, B. J., Keeler, E., and Adelstein, S. J.
Primer on certain elements of medical decision making.
New England Journal of Medicine 293:211-215, 1975.

[McNeil 78] McNeil, B. J., Weichselbaum, R. and Pauker, S. G.
Fallacy of the five-year survival in lung cancer.
New England Journal of Medicine 299:1397-1401, 1978.

[McNeil 82] McNeil, B. J., Pauker, S. G., Sox, H. C., and Tversky, A.
On the elicitation of preferences for alternative therapies.
New England Journal of Medicine 306:1259-1262, 1982.

[McWhirter 55] McWhirter, R.
Simple mastectomy and radiotherapy in treatment of breast cancer.
British Journal of Radiology 28:128-139, 1955.

[Miller 74] Miller, P. L.
A locally organized parser for spoken input.
Commun. Ass. Comput. Mach. 17:621-630, 1974.

[Miller 83a] Miller, P. L.
ATTENDING: critiquing a physician's management plan.
IEEE Transactions on Pattern Analysis and Machine Intelligence PAMI-5(5):449-461, 1983.

[Miller 83b] Miller, P. L.
Critiquing anesthetic management: the ATTENDING computer system.
Anesthesiology 58(4):362-369, 1983.

[Miller 84] Miller, P. L.
A Critiquing Approach to Expert Computer Advice: ATTENDING.
Pitman Publishing Inc., London/Boston, 1984.

[Miller 86] Miller, P. L.
Expert Critiquing Systems: Practice-Based Medical Consultation by Computer.
Springer-Verlag, New York, 1986.

[Miller, R. A. 82]
Miller, R. A., Pople, H. E., and Myers, J. D.
INTERNIST-1: an experimental computer-based diagnostic consultant for general internal medicine.
New England Journal of Medicine 307(8):468-476, 1982.
(Also appears in [Clancey 84a]).

[Moroff 83] Moroff, S. V. and Pauker, S. G.
What to do when the patient outlives the literature, or DEALE-ing with a full deck.
Medical Decision Making 3:312-338, 1983.

[Moses 84] Moses, L. E.
The series of consecutive cases as a device for assessing outcomes of intervention.
New England Journal of Medicine 311:705-710, 1984.

[Novak 83] Novak, G. S.
GLISP: A lisp-based programming system with data abstraction.
AI Magazine 4(3):37-47, 1983.

[O'Brien 81] O'Brien, P. C. and Shampoo, M. A.
Statistics for clinicians.
Mayo Clinic Proceedings 56:45-49, 126-128, 196-197, 274-276, 324-326, 393-394, 452-454, 513-515, 573-575, 639-640, 709-711, 753-756., 1981.

[Oliver 78] Oliver, N. F., Heady, J. A. and Morris, J. N. et al.
A co-operative trial in the primary prevention of ischemic heart disease using clofibrate: report from the committee of principal investigators.
British Heart Journal 40:1069-1118, 1978.

[Oliver 84] Oliver, N. F., Heady, J. A. and Morris, J. N. et al.
WHO cooperative trial on primary prevention of ischaemic heart disease with clofibrate to lower serum cholesterol: Final mortality follow-up.
Lancet 2:600-604, 1984.

[Patey 48] Patey, D. H. and Dyson, W. H.
The prognosis of carcinoma of the breast in relation to the type of operation performed.
British Journal of Cancer 2(7):7-13, 1948.

[Patil 81] Patil, R. S., Szolovits, P., and Schwartz, W. B.
Causal understanding of patient illness in medical diagnosis.
In *Proceedings of the 7th International Joint Conferences on Artificial Intelligence*, pages 893-899. Vancouver, B.C, 1981.

[Pauker 80] Pauker, S. G. and Kassirer, J. P.
The threshold approach to clincal decision making.
New England Journal of Medicine 302:1109-1117, 1980.

[Pauker 81] Pauker, S. G., and Kassirer, J. P.
Clinical decision analysis by personal computer.
Archives of Internal Medicine 141:1931-1937, 1981.

[Peters 67] Peters, M. V.
Wedge resection and irradiation.
Annals of Internal Medicine 200:144-153, 1967.

[Peters 77] Peters, M. V.
Wedge resection with or without radiation in early breast cancer.
Int. J. Radiation Oncology Biol. Phys. 2:1151-1156, 1977.

[Peto 77] Peto, R., Pike M. C., Armitage, P., Breslow, N. E., Cox, D. R., Howard, S. V., Mantel, N., McPherson, K., Peto, J., and Smith, P. G.
Design and analysis of randomized clinical trials requiring prolonged observation of each patient. II. Analysis and examples.
British Journal of Cancer 35:861-867, 1977.

[Politakis 82] Politakis, P. G.
Using empirical analysis to refine expert system knowledge bases.
PhD thesis, Computer Science Research Laboratory, Rutgers University, 1982.
Rep. No. CBM-TR-130.

[Pople 82] Pople, H.E.
Heuristic methods for imposing structure on ill-structured problems: the structuring of medical diagnostics.
Westview Press, Boulder, CO, 1982, pages 119-190, chapter 5.

[Recht 85] Recht, A., Danoff, B. S., Solin, L. J., et al.
Intraductal carcinoma of the breast: Results of treatment with excisional biopsy and irradiation.
Journal of Clinical Oncology 3:1339-1343, October, 1985.

[Rennels 86a] Rennels, G.D., Shortliffe, E.H., Stockdale, F.E. and Miller, P.L.
Reasoning from the clinical literature: the Roundsman system.
In *Proceedings of the Fifth World Congress on Medical Informatics*, pages 771-775. North-Holland, New York, October, 1986.

[Rennels 86b] Rennels, G.D., Shortliffe, E.H., Stockdale, F.E. and Miller, P.L.
Reasoning from the clinical literature: a 'distance' metric.
In *Proceedings of the AAMSI Congress 86*, pages 19-23. American Association for Medical Systems and Informatics, 1986.

[Rennels 86c] Rennels, G. D.
A computational model of reasoning from the clinical literature.
In *Proceedings of the Tenth Annual Symposium on Computer Applications in Medical Care*, pages 373-380. IEEE Computer Society Press, Washington, D.C., October, 1986.

[Rennels 86d] Rennels, G.D., Shortliffe, E.H., Stockdale, F.E. and Miller, P.L.
Updating an expert knowledge base as medical knowledge evolves: examples from oncology management.
In *Proceedings of the AAMSI Congress 87*. 1986.
(in press).

[Rennels 87a] Rennels, G. D. and Shortliffe, E. H.
Medical Advice Systems.
In Shapiro, S. (editor), *Encyclopedia of Artificial Intelligence*, . John Wiley & Sons, New York, 1987.
(in press).

[Rennels 87b] Rennels, G.D., Shortliffe, E.H., and Miller, P.L.
Choice and explanation in medical management: a multiattribute model of artifcial intelligence approaches.
Medical Decision Making 7(1):22-31, 1987.

[Rennels 87c] Rennels, G.D., Shortliffe, E.H., Stockdale, F.E. and Miller, P.L.
A computational model of reasoning from the clinical literature.
CMPB , 1987.
(in press).

[Rieger 76] Rieger, C.
An organization of knowledge for problem solving and language comprehension.
Artificial Intelligence 7:89-127, 1976.

[Rissland 85] Rissland, E. L.
Argument moves and hypotheticals.
In Charles Walter (editor), *Computing Power and Legal Reasoning*, . West Publishing Co., St. Paul, 1985.

[Rosati 75] Rosati, R. D., McNeer, J. F., Starmer, C. F., et al.
A new information system for medical practice.
Arch. Intern. Med. 135:1017-1024, 1975.

[Sager 78] Sager, N.
Natural language information formatting: the automatic conversion of texts to a structured data base.
In Yovits, M. C. and Rubinoff, M. (editor), *Advances in Computers*, pages 89-162. Academic Press, New York, 1978.
Volume 17.

[Sager 87] Sager, N.
Text processing.
In Shortliffe E. H., Wiederhold G. and Fagan L. M. (editors), *An Introduction to Medical Computer Science*, . Addison-Wesley Publishing Company, Reading, MA, expected publication 1987.
Chapter 25.

[Schreiner 84] Schreiner, J.
EXPERIPLAN: an expert system that selects statistical analyses for research studies.
SIGART Newsletter (89):27-28, 1984.
A very brief description of the system.

[Scott 77] Scott, A. C., Clancey, W. J., Davis, R., and Shortliffe, E. H.
Explanation capabilities of knowledge-based production systems.
1977.
American Journal of Computational Linguistics, Microfiche 62. (Also appears in [Buchanan 84]).

[Scura 81] Scura, Georgia and Davidoff, Frank.
Case-related use of the medical literature: clinical librarian services for improving patient care.
Journal of the American Medical Association 245(1):50-52, Jan., 1981.

[Shortliffe 75] Shortliffe, E. H. and Buchanan, B. G.
A model of inexact reasoning in medicine.
Mathematical Biosciences 23:351-379, 1975.
(Also published in [Buchanan 84]).

[Shortliffe 81] Shortliffe, E. H., Scott, A. C., Bischoff, M., Campbell, A. B. van Melle, W., and Jacobs, C.
ONCOCIN: An expert system for oncology protocol management.
In *Proceedings of the 7th International Joint Conferences on Artificial Intelligence.* IJCAI, August, 1981.
(Also published in [Buchanan 84]).

[Silverman 75] Silverman, H.
A Digitalis therapy advisor.
Project MAC TR-143, Massachusetts Institute of Technology, 1975.

[Sleeman 81] Sleeman D. H. and Brown, J. S.
Intelligent Tutoring Systems: An Overview.
Academic Press, New York, 1981.

[Spronk 84] Spronk, J. and Zionts, S.
A special issue on multiple criteria decision making.
Management Science 30(11):1265-1385, 1984.

[Sprung 84] Sprung, C. L.
The effects of high-dose corticosteroids in patients with septic shock: a prospective, controlled study.
New England Journal of Medicine 311:1137-1143, 1984.

[Stampfer 85] Stampfer, M. J., Willet, W. C., Colditz, G. A., Rosner, B., Speizer, F. E. and Hennekens, C. H.
A prospective study of postmenopausal estrogen therapy and coronary heart disease.
New England Journal of Medicine 313:1044-9, 1985.

[Stefik 86] Stefik, M. and Bobrow, D.
Object-oriented programming: Themes and variations.
AI Magazine 6(4):40-62, 1986.

[Swartout 81] Swartout, W. R.
Explaining and justifying expert consulting programs.
In *Proceedings of the 7th International Joint Conferences on Artificial Intelligence, Vancouver, B.C.*, pages 815-822. International Joint Conferences on Artificial Intelligence, August, 1981.
(Also appears in [Clancey 84a]).

[Szolovits 78] Szolovits, P. and Pauker, S.
Categorical and probabilistic reasoning in medical diagnosis.
Artificial Intelligence 11:115-144, 1978.
(Also appears in [Clancey 84a]).

[Szolovits 83] Szolovits, P. (ed.).
Artificial Intelligence In Medicine.
Westview Press, Boulder, Colorado, 1983.

[Tapley 82] Tapley, N. D., et al.
Results in patients with breast cancer treated by radical mastectomy and postoperative irradiation with no adjuvant chemotherapy.
Cancer 49:1316-1319, 1982.

[Teach 81] Teach, R. L. and Shortliffe, E. H.
An analysis of physician attitudes regarding computer-based clinical consultation systems.
Computers and Biomedical Research 14:542-558, 1981.

[Veronesi 81] Veronesi, U., Saccozzi, R. et al.
Comparing radical mastectomy with quadrantectomy, axillary dissection, and radiotherapy in patients with small cancers of the breast.
New England Journal of Medicine 305:6-11, 1981.

[Walker 81] Walker, D. E. and Hobbs, J. R.
Natural language access to medical text.
Technical Report, SRI International, March, 1981.

[Warner 72] Warner, H. R., Olmsted, C. M., and Rutherford, B. D.
HELP - a program for medical decision-making.
Computers and Biomedical Research 5:65-74, 1972.

[Warren 81] Warren, K. S.
Coping with the Biomedical Literature.
Praeger Publishers, New York, 1981.

[Weigelt 85] Weigelt, J. A., Norcross, J. F., Borman, K. R. and Snyder, W. H.
Early steroid therapy for respiratory failure.
Archives of Surgery 120:536-540, 1985.

[Weiner 80] Weiner, J. L.
BLAH, A system which explains its reasoning.
Artificial Intelligence 15:19-48, 1980.

[Weiss 78] Weiss, S. M., Kulikowski, C. A., Amarel, S. and Safir, A.
A model-based method for computer-aided medical decision making.
Artificial Intelligence 11:145-172, 1978.
(Also published in [Clancey 84a]).

[Weiss 81] Weiss, S. M., Kulikowski, C. A., and Galen, R. S.
Developing microprocessor-based expert models for instrument interpretation.
In *Proceedings of the Seventh International Joint Conferences on Artificial Intelligence*, pages 853-855. 1981.
(also published in [Clancey 84a]).

[Wellman 85] Wellman, M. P.
Reasoning About Preference Models.
Master's thesis, Massachusetts Institute of Technology, 1985.

[Weyl 75] Weyl, S., Fries, J., Wiederhold, G., and Germano, F.
A modular self-describing clinical databank system.
Computers and Biomedical Research 8:279-293, 1975.

[Wilson 85] Wilson, P. W., Garrison, R. J. and Castelli, W. P.
Postmenopausal estrogen use, cigarette smoking, and cardiovascular morbidity in women over 50.
New England Journal of Medicine 313:1038-43, 1985.

[Winston 75] Winston, P. H.
Learning structural descriptions from examples.
In P.H. Winston (editor), *The Psychology of Computer Vision,* .
McGraw-Hill Book Company, New York, 1975.

[Woods 70] Woods, W. A.
Transition network grammars for natural language analysis.
Commun. Ass. Comput. Mach. 13:591-606, 1970.

[Yu 79] Yu, V. L., Fagan, L. M., Wraith, S. M., Clancey, W. J. Scott, A. C. Hannigan, J. F., Blum, R. L., Buchanan, B. G. and Cohen, S. N.
Antimicrobial selection by a computer: A blinded evaluation by infectious disease experts.
Journal of the American Medical Association 242(12):1279-1282, 1979.
also published in [Buchanan 84].

Index

Lecture Notes in Medical Informatics

Vol. 23: Selected Topics in Image Science. Edited by O. Nalcioglu and Z.-H. Cho. IX, 308 pages. 1984.

Vol. 24: Medical Informatics Europe 1984. Proceedings, 1984. Edited by F.H. Roger, J.L. Willems, R. O'Moore and B. Barber. XXVII, 778 pages. 1984.

Vol. 25: Medical Informatics Europe 1985. Edited by F.H. Roger, P. Grönroos, R. Tervo-Pellikka and R. O'Moore. XVII, 823 pages. 1985.

Vol. 26: Methodical Problems in Early Detection Programmes. Proceedings, 1983. Edited by E. Walter and A. Neiß. VIII, 198 pages. 1985.

Vol. 27: E. Mergenthaler, Textbank Systems. VI, 177 pages. 1985.

Vol. 28: Objective Medical Decision Making. Proceedings, 1985. Edited by D.D. Tsiftsis. VII, 229 pages. 1986.

Vol. 29: System Analysis of Ambulatory Care in Selected Countries. Edited by P.L. Reichertz, R. Engelbrecht and U. Piccolo. VI, 197 pages. 1986.

Vol. 30: Present Status of Computer Support in Ambulatory Care. Edited by P.L. Reichertz, R. Engelbrecht and U. Piccolo. VIII, 241 pages. 1987.

Vol. 31: S.J. Duckett, Operations Research for Health Planning and Administration. III, 165 pages. 1987.

Vol. 32: G.D. Rennels, A Computational Model of Reasoning from the Clinical Literature. XV, 230 pages. 1987.

GPSR Compliance

The European Union's (EU) General Product Safety Regulation (GPSR) is a set of rules that requires consumer products to be safe and our obligations to ensure this.

If you have any concerns about our products, you can contact us on ProductSafety@springernature.com

In case Publisher is established outside the EU, the EU authorized representative is:

Springer Nature Customer Service Center GmbH
Europaplatz 3
69115 Heidelberg, Germany

Batch number: 10704763

Printed by Printforce, the Netherlands